Preparing for the ACSM Health/Fitness Instructor Certification Examination

Second Edition

Larry D. Isaacs, PhD
Roberta L. Pohlman, PhD

Wright State University
Dayton, Ohio

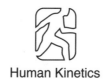

Human Kinetics

Library of Congress Cataloging-in-Publication Data

Isaacs, Larry D. (Larry David), 1949-
Preparing for the ACSM health/fitness instructor certification
examination / Larry D. Isaacs, Roberta L. Pohlman.--2nd ed.
p. ; cm.
Includes bibliographical references.
ISBN 0-7360-4240-7
1. Personal trainers--Certification--United
States--Examinations--Study guides.
[DNLM: 1. Physical Education and Training--United States--Examination
Questions. 2. Certification--United States--Examination Questions.]
I. Pohlman, Roberta, 1951- II. American College of Sports Medicine. III.
Title.
GV428.7.I73 2004
613.7'11'076--dc22

2003019593

ISBN: 0-7360-4240-7

Copyright © 2004 by Larry D. Isaacs and Roberta L. Pohlman

The Web addresses cited in this text were current as of August 15, 2003, unless otherwise noted.

Acquisitions Editor: Michael S. Bahrke, PhD; **Developmental Editor:** Jeff King; **Assistant Editor:** Anne Cole; **Copyeditor:** Jennifer Davis; **Proofreader:** Kim Thoren; **Permission Manager:** Dalene Reeder; **Graphic Designer:** Fred Starbird; **Graphic Artist:** Kathleen Boudreau-Fuoss; **Cover Designer:** Keith Blomberg; **Printer:** United Graphics

Printed in the United States of America   10   9   8   7   6   5   4   3   2   1

Human Kinetics
Web site: www.HumanKinetics.com

United States: Human Kinetics
P.O. Box 5076
Champaign, IL 61825-5076
800-747-4457
e-mail: humank@hkusa.com

Canada: Human Kinetics
475 Devonshire Road Unit 100
Windsor, ON N8Y 2L5
800-465-7301 (in Canada only)
e-mail: orders@hkcanada.com

Europe: Human Kinetics
107 Bradford Road, Stanningley
Leeds LS28 6AT, United Kingdom
+44 (0) 113 255 5665
e-mail: hk@hkeurope.com

Australia: Human Kinetics
57A Price Avenue, Lower Mitcham
South Australia 5062
08 8277 1555
e-mail: liaw@hkaustralia.com

New Zealand: Human Kinetics
Division of Sports Distributors NZ Ltd.
P.O. Box 300 226 Albany
North Shore City, Auckland
0064 9 448 1207
e-mail: blairc@hknewz.com

To my children,
Brooke and Timothy;
to the memory of my loving parents,
Linwood and Gracie;
and to the memory of my feline friends,
Lucy, Burt, and Ernie

Larry D. Isaacs

To my friends and family
for their love and support

Roberta L. Pohlman

Contents

Preface

*P*reparing for the ACSM Health/Fitness Instructor Certification Examination, Second Edition,* is the only comprehensive preparatory text of its kind written specifically for the purpose of preparing you to pass this highly sought-after certification offered through the prestigious American College of Sports Medicine (ACSM). In fact, ACSM certifications are considered the gold standard among exercise science professionals.

To help you get the most from this preparatory text, we have divided it into three parts. In part I, we carefully walk you through the certification process (chapter 1). Here you will learn about the eligibility criteria for certification, registration procedures for the certification examination, and the general structure of both the written and practical portions of the certification process. Perhaps most important, we then provide detailed information about both the written (chapter 2) and the practical (chapter 3) examinations. Here we describe the 10 content areas that the written certification examination covers and even tell you approximately how many questions you can expect in each area. In addition, we highlight test-taking suggestions and special precautions that will undoubtedly improve your test score by reducing your chance of making an unnecessary error. We then describe, in detail, the three aspects of the practical examination (chapter 3). Not only will you learn the specific tasks that you will likely be required to perform at each of the three practical examination stations, but you will also have a list of preparatory strategies specifically geared to this aspect of the certification examination, including tips on how to get the practical experience necessary to pass this part of the ACSM Health/Fitness Instructor certification examination.

In part II, you will find nearly 600 practice study questions. More specifically, for each of the 10 examination content areas, there is an entire chapter of study questions. These study questions are similar to the questions you are likely to encounter on your written certification examination. And, perhaps most important, each practice study question is designed to assess your knowledge, skills, and abilities (KSAs) as used by ACSM to describe the minimal competencies necessary to obtain ACSM certification. Each chapter of study questions ends with a detailed answer sheet. On the answer sheet, you will find the answer to each study question as well as a reference to a source (with page number) where you can find more information about the concept. Furthermore, the specific ACSM KSA being measured by each question is identified. This arrangement will not only save you time by referring you to important study materials but will also allow you to pinpoint specific areas of weakness within each of the 10 examination (KSA) categories. Part II ends with two special chapters, each addressing a special form of questioning to which you will need to respond during the certification process. More specifically, in chapter 14 you will learn how to solve metabolic equations, and in chapter 15 you will learn how to answer questions when information is presented in the form of a case study. These chapters will help prepare you for questions posed during both the written and the practical portions of the examination.

The third and final part of this preparatory text is made up of appendixes. Appendix A is a complete practice Health/Fitness Instructor certification examination containing 115 questions. This practice examination was designed to simulate the actual written examination in terms of length, time limit (three hours), and question emphasis (i.e., number of questions from each KSA examination category). When taking this practice examination, be sure to record your answers on the blank score sheet provided in appendix B. This preparatory text ends with a specially designed answer sheet (appendix C) for the practice examination and a practice examination profile sheet (appendix D). The first part of this answer sheet simply provides a list of answers (#1-115) for the practice examination. However, on the second portion of the answer sheet, the answers are classified according to the 10 KSA categories. This special breakdown will allow you to fill in the profile sheet to identify specific areas of strength and weakness. Obviously, you will want to devote additional study time to identified areas of weakness before attempting ACSM certification.

In summary, this preparatory text, *Preparing for the ACSM Health/ Fitness Instructor Certification Examination, Second Edition,* will help you develop your confidence in test-taking strategies for successfully obtaining ACSM certification.

List of Abbreviations

ADP	andenosine diphosphate
ATP	adenosine triphosphate
AV	atrioventricular
a-$\bar{V}O_2$ diff	arteriovenous oxygen difference
BMI	body mass index
BP	blood pressure
Ca^{++}	calcium
CAD	coronary artery disease
CHO	carbohydrate
CP	creatine phosphate
CPR	cardiopulmonary resuscitation
CRF	cardiorespiratory function
DBP	diastolic blood pressure
DOMS	delayed onset of muscle soreness
ECG	electrocardiogram
EMS	emergency medical system
FIT	frequency, intensity, time
GXT	graded exercise test
HDL-C	high-density lipoprotein-cholesterol
HR	heart rate
HRR	heart rate reserve
IDDM	insulin-dependent diabetes mellitus
kcal	kilocalories
LDL-C	low-density lipoprotein-cholesterol
MET	metabolic equivalent
mmHg	millimeters of mercury
MVC	maximal voluntary contraction
O_2	oxygen
OBLA	onset of blood lactate accumulation

PC	phosphocreatine
PVC	premature ventricular contraction
PWC	physical work capacity
Q	cardiac output
RM	repetition maximum
ROM	range of motion
RPE	rate of perceived exertion
SA	sinoatrial node
SBP	systolic blood pressure
SV	stroke volume
TC	total cholesterol
USDA	United States Department of Agriculture
VLDL-C	very low density lipoprotein-cholesterol
$V_E/\dot{V}O_2$	ventilatory equivalent
$\dot{V}O_2max$	maximal oxygen consumption

PART

I

About the Examination

CHAPTER 1

Understanding and Preparing for ACSM Certification

Congratulations! You have chosen to become certified by an organization considered to be the gold standard among professionals in the fields of health, fitness, and cardiac rehabilitation. The American College of Sports Medicine (ACSM) certification tracks, as you will read, are designed to increase your competency in your specific area of interest. When you receive your ACSM certification, you will know that you are among an elite group of professionals internationally recognized for their knowledge, skills, and abilities in the fields of health and fitness. Let's begin by examining the ACSM certification process.

ACSM CERTIFICATION

Certification through ACSM is organized around two distinct tracks. The Health/Fitness Track, the primary emphasis in this text, consists of certifications (Exercise Group Leader, Health/Fitness Instructor, Health/Fitness Director) that are geared toward individuals who wish to provide program leadership to apparently healthy individuals and, in some cases, individuals with controlled disease. These programs are primarily preventive in nature. In contrast, certifications within the Clinical Track (Exercise Specialist, Program Director) involve working both with individuals at high risk of disease and individuals who have known diseases. Also within the clinical track is ACSM's newest certification, Clinical Exercise Physiology (ACSM, 2002).

In this text, we will focus exclusively on the second level of certification within the Health/Fitness Track, namely that of Health/Fitness

Instructor. Note that certification at an advanced level requires the candidate to possess the knowledge base and skills associated with that level of certification as well as the knowledge base and skills required of any level below that level of certification. Therefore, certification at the level of Health/Fitness Instructor requires the candidate to demonstrate a command of the knowledge base and skills at both the level of Exercise Group Leader and the level of Health/Fitness Instructor.

Eligibility Criteria for Health/Fitness Instructor Certification

Minimum requirements to register for the ACSM Health/Fitness Instructor certification examination include the following:

1. Obtain a 2-year, 4-year, or master's degree from an accredited college or university in a health-related field to include exercise science, kinesiology, athletic training, physical education, exercise physiology, human performance, biology, and sport management. Verification may be required by transcript or copy of the degree.

OR

2. Current enrollment as a junior or higher from an accredited college or university in a health-related field.

OR

3. Have a minimum of 900 hours of practical experience in a fitness setting,

and

4. Possess up-to-date CPR certification.

Obtaining an Application

Regardless of your time frame for obtaining certification, we recommend that you request an application as soon as possible. You can obtain an application by contacting the ACSM Certification Resource Center at 800-486-5643. Ask for the current ACSM Certification Resource Catalog. This catalog will contain an application, a list of dates and locations of planned certification sites, and a list of recommended publications for study. If you prefer, this information can be obtained online from the following URL: www.LWW.com/acsmcrc.

Registering for the Certification Examination

When completing the Health/Fitness Instructor application, you will note that you need to make several decisions. More specifically, you will need to select a preferred certification site and date as well as an alternative in case your first choice is not available. We suggest that to improve your chances of gaining admission to your preferred site you submit the application as soon as possible. Also note that many of the certification sites offer a precertification workshop (see discussion later in this chapter). If you plan to attend the workshop before the certification examination, you must note this on the application. You will also be required to sign a statement verifying up-to-date CPR certification and to confirm that you have met the entire minimum requirement for taking this level of certification examination.

After completing the application, you should make two photocopies of it. Keep one for your records and mail the original, along with one photocopy and the appropriate fees (check, money order, MasterCard or VISA), to the address listed at the bottom of the application. Please note that this address is that of the ACSM National Center in Indianapolis, Indiana, *not* that of the ACSM Resource Center from which you obtained the application.

TEST STRUCTURE AND ADMINISTRATION

The ACSM Health/Fitness Instructor certification examination has two components: a written examination consisting of approximately 115 multiple-choice questions and a 60-minute practical examination (3 stations, each 20 minutes in length). Each of these certification components is designed to test the knowledge, skills, and abilities (KSAs) that a certified Health/Fitness Instructor needs in order to perform his or her duties. These KSAs are organized around the 10 categories outlined in table 1.1 (see also ACSM, 2000, p. 328).

The practical examination will also require you to demonstrate knowledge and skill by performing such tasks as identifying and collecting anthropometric data, including skinfolds and circumferential assessments; demonstrating flexibility and strength exercises; administering

Table 1.1   KSA Categories

Anatomy and Biomechanics
Exercise Physiology
Human Development and Aging
Pathophysiology and Risk Factors
Human Behavior and Psychology
Health Appraisal and Fitness Testing
Safety, Injury Prevention, and Emergency Care
Exercise Programming
Nutrition and Weight Management
Program Administration and Management

tests of flexibility and muscular endurance; and preparing to administer, as well as administering, selected aspects of a physical work capacity (PWC) test. In chapters 2 and 3, we explain the details of each of these examinations and offer practical advice on how to prepare for each.

What to Expect on Test Day

Knowing what to expect on test day can greatly reduce test anxiety. Note the following points about the test-day procedures:

1. Arrive at the predetermined certification site at least 30 minutes before the time the test is scheduled to begin. This holds true for both the written and the practical examinations.

2. Upon checking in, you will be required to show positive proof of identification by producing a driver's license or passport. Anyone unable to provide one of these forms of identification *will not* be allowed to take the certification examination.

3. Bring several number 2 pencils and a calculator to the written examination. The calculator must be of the simplest variety; *no programmable calculators are allowed.*

4. At the designated examination time, the written certification examination will be distributed to each candidate. The exami-

nation will be in an individually sealed envelope. You are *not* to open the envelope until instructed to do so. From the time this instruction is given you will be allowed three hours to complete the written examination.

5. When turning in the completed examination, you will be required to place the test questions, as well as your score sheet, back into the envelope. The envelope will be sealed and a special label will be placed across the envelope's sealed tab. To complete the process, you will be asked to place your signature on this label.

6. With regard to the practical examination, a special briefing session is typically scheduled the day before the examination. At this time, you will be given an explanation of the exam process and a schedule confirming the time of your examination. You will also have the opportunity to familiarize yourself with the equipment that will be used during the practical examination. This is especially helpful for candidates who have not participated in a precertification workshop.

Scoring

Both the written and the practical examinations are scored at the ACSM National Office. A passing score for the written examination is determined by the ACSM Certification Subcommittee on the basis of normative data.

Even though the practical examination is evaluated on the basis of your performance at each of three examination stations (see chapter 3), your score will be calculated as a function of your overall performance. While questions on the practical examination are differentially weighted, you cannot fail this portion of the certification process by missing any one question. Once again, the score needed to pass the practical examination is determined annually by the ACSM Certification Subcommittee (ACSM, 2003).

Notification of Results

Within four to six weeks you will receive your test results by mail for both the written and the practical examinations. Results of both examinations are reported as pass/fail and you will be told of the number of questions which you answered correctly within each KSA category. Additionally, candidates who fail the practical examination will receive a detailed analysis based on KSAs associated with selected questions from the practical examination. The purpose of this analysis is to give you information regarding personal strengths and weaknesses identified during the practical examination. To receive certification, you must obtain a passing score on both the written and the practical examinations.

Retesting Procedures

If you fail either the written or the practical examination, you will be required to retest on the component you did not pass. All the registration procedures described earlier also hold true for the retest. We *strongly recommend* that you use the information presented on the notification of results to prepare for retesting. You must complete retesting within one year. If you do not meet this requirement, you will need to begin the certification process again.

PREPARING FOR CERTIFICATION

Preparation is the key to successfully passing the Health/Fitness Instructor certification examination. In this section we offer advice to help you prepare effectively.

Precertification Workshops

As previously mentioned, three- to four-day precertification workshops are offered at many of the certification examination sites. These workshops consist of approximately 20 hours of lecture covering all of the vital KSA categories. In addition, at a workshop you will have ample time to practice the tasks you will need to perform during the practical examination. More specifically, practical sessions include physical work capacity testing using a cycle ergometer; body composition, flexibility, and strength assessment; and health and fitness consultations. We highly recommend this preparatory experience.

SUGGESTIONS FOR USING THIS PREPARATORY TEXT

Now that you have a better understanding of the certification process, you should be ready and eager to begin preparing. Here are a few suggestions on how you can best use this text as you begin the preparatory process:

- Since ACSM summarizes important information in table form, you should obtain copies of, and memorize, the materials listed in table 1.2. This is critical information. In addition to this text, we also suggest the sources listed in table 1.3.
- Begin by reviewing the ACSM KSAs beginning on page 328 in the sixth edition of *ACSM's Guidelines for Exercise Testing and Prescription* (ACSM, 2000). These numbered KSAs describe in detail the

Table 1.2   Important Tables to Study in Preparing for ACSM Health/Fitness Instructor Certification

Tables to study	Page number*
Coronary Artery Disease Risk Factor Thresholds	24
Initial ACSM Risk Stratification	26
ACSM Recommendations for Medical Exam and Exercise Testing Prior to Participation and Physician Supervision of Exercise Tests	27
Informed Consent (Sample Form)	53
Standardized Description of Skinfold Sites and Procedures	65
Rating of Perceived Exertion Scales	79
YMCA Cycle Ergometry Protocol	75
General Procedures for Submaximal Testing of Cardiorespiratory Endurance Using a Cycle Ergometer	72
Push-Up Test Procedures	84
Trunk Flexion Test Procedures	87
Absolute and Relative Indications for Termination of an Exercise Test	50
General Indications for Stopping an Exercise Test in Low-Risk Adults	80
Major Signs or Symptoms Suggestive of CV and Pulmonary Disease	25

*From ACSM, 2000, *ACSM's guidelines for exercise testing and prescription,* 6th ed. (Philadelphia: Lippincott Williams & Wilkins).

Table 1.3   Other Useful Sources for Study

Key Sources of Information
ACSM. (2001). *ACSM's resource manual for guidelines for exercise testing and prescription* (4th ed.). Philadelphia: Lippincott Williams & Wilkins.
ACSM. (2000). *ACSM's guidelines for exercise testing and prescription* (6th ed.). Philadelphia: Lippincott Williams and Wilkins.
Baechle, T.R., & Earle, R.W. (Ed.). (2000). *Essentials of strength training and conditioning* (2nd ed.). Champaign, IL: Human Kinetics.
Hall, S.J. (2003). *Basic biomechanics* (4th ed.). Boston: McGraw-Hill.
Howley, E.T., & Franks, B.D. (2003). *Health fitness instructor's handbook* (4th ed.). Champaign, IL: Human Kinetics.
McArdle, W.D., Katch, F.I., & Katch. V.I. (2001). *Exercise physiology: Energy, nutrition, and human performance* (5th ed.). Philadelphia: Lippincott Williams & Williams.
Nieman, D.C. (2003). Exercise testing and prescription (5th ed.). Boston: McGraw-Hill.
Seeley, R.R., Stephens, T.D., & Tate, P. (2003). *Anatomy & physiology* (6th ed.). Boston: McGraw-Hill.

competencies you will be required to exhibit in order to receive your Health/Fitness Instructor certification. Then, note that as you work through this book, you will find an answer key at the end of each study-question chapter (chapters 4-13) specific to a KSA. This key contains the answer to each study question, a KSA number (note that you will be responsible for all KSA's beginning with the numbers 1 and 2) from *ACSM's Guidelines for Exercise Testing and Prescription* (ACSM, 2000) to help you identify the objective of the question and one or more appropriate references, with page numbers, for further study.

• Divide your study time into manageable units. You can accomplish this by concentrating on one KSA category at a time.

• In appendix A, we have supplied a practice Health/Fitness Instructor certification examination. You can use this examination in one of two ways. One option is to use it as a pretest to help you identify your strengths and weaknesses within each of the KSA categories. Another option is to work through this study guide by answering the study questions presented in chapters 4 through 15 and then use the practice examination as a posttest.

REFERENCES

ACSM. (2003). *ACSM certification resource center catalog.* Philadelphia: Lippincott Williams & Wilkins.

ACSM. (2002). *ACSM's resources for clinical exercise physiology.* Philadelphia: Lippincott Williams & Wilkins.

ACSM. (2000). *ACSM's guidelines for exercise testing and prescription* (6th ed.). Philadelphia: Lippincott Williams & Wilkins.

2

The Written Examination

The written examination is designed to assess your ability to recall and apply facts as defined by the ACSM KSAs. These KSAs are located in appendix F in *ACSM's Guidelines for Exercise Testing and Prescription, Sixth Edition* (ACSM, 2000).

EXAMINATION FORMAT AND NUMBER OF QUESTIONS

The written examination consists of approximately 115 multiple-choice questions. There are approximately 15 questions on this exam that will not be graded. Each multiple-choice question will consist of a stem (the question) followed by four (*a-d*) or five (*a-e*) possible answers (options). Table 2.1 indicates the number of questions that you are likely to encounter in each of the examination categories.

Time Limit and Scoring

You will have a maximum of three hours to take the written examination. As a general rule, you should spend no more than one minute answering any one question. Questions that require you to perform mathematical calculations—most notably those that require you to solve metabolic equations as discussed in chapter 14—are an exception. The overall point is that you should not spend too much time pondering any single question. Instead, leave a blank for any question that gives you trouble and plan to return to it after you have answered all the other questions.

Table 2.1   Potential Number of Questions From Each KSA Category

Examination category	Number of questions*
Anatomy and Biomechanics	8
Exercise Physiology	20
Human Development and Aging	8
Pathophysiology and Risk Factors	10
Human Behavior and Psychology	5
Health Appraisal and Fitness Testing	10
Safety, Injury Prevention, and Emergency Care	5
Exercise Programming	22
Nutrition and Weight Management	6
Program Administration and Management	6
Metabolic Calculations	10**

*Potential number of questions as reported by ACSM (2003). Visit www.LWW. com/acsmcrc/ hfinstr.html for more information.
**Within the H/FI certification examination questions, approximately ten will require you to calculate a metabolic equation.

Adapted, by permission, from American College of Sports Medicine, 2003, *ACSM certification category* (Philadelphia: Lippincott Williams and Wilkins). Available on www.lww.com/acsmer/ hfinstr.html

Each multiple-choice question has only one correct answer, so your answer will be scored as either correct or incorrect. There is no penalty for guessing, and all questions are of equal weight.

TEST-TAKING SUGGESTIONS

Here are a few suggestions to help improve your score:

- Read each question carefully, taking time to underline any key terms.
- Attempt, in your own mind, to answer each question before looking at the choices. (Use your hand to cover up the choices.)

- If your answer is not among the choices given, attempt to eliminate answers that you are confident are incorrect. This will greatly increase your odds of selecting (or in some cases guessing) the correct answer.
- If you are uncertain about an answer, skip that question and move on. However, place a large mark beside the question so that you can easily come back to it later on.
- Since you will not be penalized for guessing, never leave a question blank. Always select one of the multiple-choice answers.
- Check your answer sheet to be sure you have not inadvertently left out a response.

Test-Taking Precautions

At one time or another we have all been exposed to a poorly constructed teacher-made test in which an answer is so obvious that it nearly jumps off the test and onto the answer sheet. Don't expect this to be the case with your written certification examination. Indeed, the ACSM Health/Fitness Instructor written certification examination is a skillfully constructed assessment instrument. Outlined here are a couple of special precautions that you should keep in mind to improve your score.

Be aware that a number of the questions on your written certification examination will require multiple thought processes. For example, compare the thought processes associated with these two questions:

_____ 1. The amount of blood ejected from the left ventricle with each beat is referred to as
   a. cardiac index
   b. cardiac output
   c. ejection fraction
   d. stroke volume

_____ 2. Mary is a 40-year-old female with a resting HR of 78 beats per minute and a maximal HR of 183 beats per minute. Using the HRR method, identify Mary's target HR when intensity is established as 70 percent of HRR.
   a. 126 beats per minute
   b. 142 beats per minute
   c. a 15-second pulse of 38 beats
   d. a 10-second pulse of 15 beats

The correct answer to the first question is *d*, stroke volume. This first question required just one simple thought process. In comparison, the second question is more difficult because it requires you to carry out several mental functions to derive the correct response. You will encounter both kinds of questions on the examination, so beware.

Let's examine the thought processes needed to correctly answer the second question. First, you had to recall the HRR, or Karvonen, formula. You then had to extract the important information from the question to substitute into the formula (HR max = 183 beats per minute; resting HR = 78 beats per minute; 70 percent exercise intensity). You then mathematically solved the formula. You could see quickly that your answer of 152 beats per minute was not listed among the possible answers. You then had to convert responses *c* and *d* to beats per minute. Now you could see that *c*, a 15-second pulse of 38 beats, was the correct answer (4 × 38 = 152 beats per minute).

Furthermore, had you selected the inappropriate rule-of-thumb formula (HR max = 220 – age), you would have incorrectly selected answer *a* (220 – 40 = 180 × .70 = 126 beats per minute). As should be evident, the test writers for this examination are well aware of the mistakes people most commonly make on a given question. This knowledge allows them to include such incorrect responses among the available options. For this reason, don't rush into selecting an answer thinking that you must be correct because it appears among the possible responses. Instead, take your time and think through the logic underlying each question.

Pay close attention to units of measure and the locations of decimal points. You may confront a list of potential answers that at first glance look similar but in reality are different. An example of this is a question with the answers 25 L, 2.5 L, .25 L, 25 ml, 2.5 ml, and .25 ml.

After you have completed the entire written examination, revisit any unanswered questions. Then, if time remains, it is advisable to check over any questions that required you to perform mathematical calculations. However, avoid the temptation to change previously answered questions without thinking through your rationale for making the change.

REFERENCES

ACSM. (2003). *ACSM certification resource center catalog*. Philadelphia: Lippincott Williams & Wilkins.

ACSM. (2000). *ACSM's guidelines for exercise testing and prescription* (6th ed.). Philadelphia: Lippincott Williams & Wilkins.

CHAPTER 3

The Practical Examination

While the written examination is specifically designed to test your knowledge of the ACSM KSAs, the practical examination is designed to test your ability to apply this knowledge as would be required in a real-world setting. In other words, the emphasis of the practical examination is not only on knowing what to do but also on being able to carry out a defined task appropriately. In this chapter, we discuss the format of the practical examination and describe, in some detail, tasks that you should practice and master before taking your certification examination.

EXAMINATION FORMAT

The practical exam is divided into three examination stations. Certification candidates are randomly assigned an initial station and rotate through the remaining two. Upon entering an examination station, you will be greeted by an ACSM-certified examiner. The examiner is trained to ask a series of prepared questions or describe a scenario to which you must respond. You will be allotted a maximum of 20 minutes at each of the three stations.

When responding to an examiner's question or scenario, you must adhere to one very important assumption: While your examiner will be knowledgeable and well trained, you must nevertheless gear your responses as if you were communicating with a client who possesses little knowledge of the subject matter in question.

Three Practical Examination Stations

Here is a brief description of each of the three practical examination stations, along with a list of tasks you may be asked to perform.

Station 1

The first station is designed to assess your knowledge and abilities in the areas of anthropometric measurement, body composition assessment, and demonstration of upper- and lower-body flexibility exercises. To prepare for this part of the examination you should be able to do the following:

- Identify standardized skinfold assessment sites as outlined on page 65 of *ACSM's Guidelines for Exercise Testing and Prescription, Sixth Edition* (2000). Your examiner may name a specific site, requiring you to appropriately identify and assess this area using standard skinfold calipers.

- Identify standardized circumferential sites as outlined on page 63 of *ACSM's Guidelines* (2000) and pages 101 to 103 of *ACSM's Resource Manual for Guidelines for Exercise Testing and Prescription, Fourth Edition* (2001). Your examiner may name a specific site, requiring you to appropriately identify and assess this area using a Gulick (tension-regulated) tape.

- Demonstrate and administer the sit-and-reach test protocol, adhering to the standards outlined on page 87 of *ACSM's Guidelines* (2000).

- Describe and demonstrate a flexibility exercise for a specific muscle group. Here your examiner may name a muscle group, requiring you to select and demonstrate an appropriate flexibility exercise. We suggest that you consult the chapter titled "Stretching and Warm-Up" by Holcomb, which you will find in chapter 16 of *Essentials of Strength Training and Conditioning, Second Edition* (Baechle & Earle, 2000). Another excellent source to consult is *Sport Stretch, Second Edition* (Alter, 1998).

Station 2

The second station is designed to assess your knowledge, skills, and abilities with respect to demonstrating, evaluating, and supervising strength and conditioning exercises using one's own body weight, as well as a variety of equipment, including dumbbells, free weights, and a stability ball. To help prepare for this second practical station, we would suggest that you be able to do the following:

- Demonstrate various resistance-training exercises for all the major muscle groups. We suggest that you consult Baechle & Earle (2000), especially chapter 17. This source describes and illustrates 32 strength-training exercises, highlighting the body region being trained. Another excellent source is Delavier's *Strength Training Anatomy* (2001). This text is well illustrated and highlights the major muscles used in performing nearly all of the most frequently used strength training exercises.

- Explain and demonstrate the push-up endurance test protocol as discussed on page 84 in *ACSM's Guidelines* (2000). As with any muscular resistance activity, keep a watchful eye on the participant to ensure that he or she does not exhibit breath-holding. You must also insist that the person maintain correct form and technique at all times when performing any resistance-training exercise.

Station 3

The third station is designed to assess your ability to prepare for and administer a submaximal PWC test performed on a Monark cycle ergometer. You will be required to administer the YMCA Cycle Ergometry Protocol, which is reproduced in *ACSM's Guidelines* (2000, p. 75). Be sure to conduct the test in accordance with the established guidelines outlined on page 72 of the *ACSM's Guidelines* (2000). At this station, you must be prepared to do the following:

- Appropriately explain an informed consent form. In your explana-tion, be sure to address each of the seven important components contained in an informed consent form. Consult *ACSM's Guidelines* (2000), page 53, for a generic informed consent form.

- Explain to a client the purpose for using, and describe how to use, the rating of perceived exertion (RPE) scale. Consult *ACSM's Guidelines* (2000), page 79, for an explanation and a copy of the RPE scale.

- Properly adjust a cycle ergometer in preparation for an exercise test. Pay particular attention to point 3 of the "Standardized Guidelines for Submaximal Cardiovascular Evaluation" on page 72 in the *ACSM's Guidelines* (2000). Be prepared to demonstrate how you can adjust the ergometer's seat to accomplish a five-degree bend at the knee joint when the pedal is at the endpoint in the downstroke.

- Obtain a preexercise HR.
- Obtain a preexercise BP (see American Heart Association, 1987).
- Adjust workload at the appropriate time and to the appropriate level (ACSM, 2000, p. 75).
- Measure HR, BP, and RPE at the appropriate times (ACSM, 2000, p. 72. See points 4, 5, and 6).
- Know when to terminate the test (see ACSM, 2000, p. 80).
- Keep a watchful eye on the participant, looking for inappropriate changes in appearance or the presence of abnormal symptoms.
- Periodically ask the participant, "Are you feeling okay?"

SPECIAL ARRANGEMENTS FOR INDIVIDUALS WITH DISABILITIES

As should now be evident, the practical examination requires the candidate to demonstrate various tasks accurately. ACSM recognizes that individuals with disabilities may not be physically capable of performing some of the certification tasks. Therefore, ACSM will make special arrangements for individuals with disabilities so as not to exclude, segregate, or treat them differently from any other certification candidate. If you have a disability that requires special auxiliary aids or services as identified in the Americans with Disability Act, you should contact the ACSM National Office (317-637-9200) and request a copy of the form "A Special Note for the Disabled." On this form, you will be asked to describe your disability and any special equipment or situational needs. You should then return the form, along with written verification of your disability from a qualified professional, to the ACSM National Office no later than 30 days (and preferably as soon as possible) before your workshop and/or certification date. Copies of the form and letter of disability verification should also be sent directly to your scheduled workshop or certification site. ACSM will notify you of any approved arrangements.

PREPARATION STRATEGIES

As mentioned in the introduction, it is important that you practice and master the tasks outlined in this chapter before attempting certification. We suggest that approximately three to six months before the certification examination you make arrangements to practice these tasks under the supervision of a trained professional. Volunteer internships are frequently available in community fitness programs and in college-, corporate-, and hospital-sponsored fitness programs.

While working under the supervision of a trained professional as you practice, you should strive to collect anthropometric measurements, both skinfold and circumferential measurements, on 75 to 100 individuals. To check your accuracy, ask the trained professional to perform these measurements also, and compare your measurements with theirs.

Other important ways you can prepare include leading a group exercise class through both a warm-up and a cool-down cycle, administering the sit-and-reach test and the push-up endurance test to at least 75 individuals, explaining and demonstrating appropriate resistance-training exercises to at least 50 individuals, and administering at least 50 submaximal cycle ergometry tests using the protocols outlined in this chapter. With appropriate practice, your confidence will increase and your anxiety regarding this phase of the certification examination will diminish.

REFERENCES

ACSM. (2001). *ACSM's resource manual for guidelines for exercise testing and prescription* (4th ed.). Philadelphia: Lippincott Williams & Wilkins.

ACSM. (2000). *ACSM's guidelines for exercise testing and prescription* (6th ed.). Philadelphia: Lippincott Williams & Wilkins.

Alter, M.J. (1998). *Sport stretch* (2nd ed.). Champaign, IL: Human Kinetics.

American Heart Association. (1987). *Recommendations for human blood pressure determination by sphygmomanometer*. Dallas: American Heart Association.

Baechle, T.R., & Earle, R.W. (Eds.) (2000). *Essentials of strength training and conditioning* (2nd ed.). Champaign, IL: Human Kinetics.

Delavier, F. (2001). *Strength training anatomy*. Champaign, IL: Human Kinetics.

PART

II

Examination Study Questions

CHAPTER

4

Anatomy and Biomechanics

This ACSM KSA category, Anatomy and Biomechanics, consists of 20 objectives, each containing multiple elements. While you may have only eight questions from this category on your certification examination, we have constructed 92 practice questions to help you prepare for such a major content area. You should consult the textbooks cited at the end of this chapter because they will provide you with the knowledge base you will need to pass this KSA category.

PRACTICE QUESTIONS

Instructions: Each question is followed by either four or five possible answers. Select the *best* answer to each question.

___ 1. The sphenoid bone, facial bones, and vertebrae are classified as what type of bone?

    a. long

    b. flat

    c. short

    d. irregular

___ 2. What is indicated by an ossified epiphyseal plate located between the diaphysis and epiphysis of a long bone?

    a. The bone can no longer increase in length.

    b. The area around the plate is dead.

c. The diameter of the bone will decrease.

d. The bone is in a stage of growth.

____ 3. In mature bone,

a. cancellous and compact bone are fully developed

b. the epiphyseal plate is now the epiphyseal line

c. the only cartilage present is articular cartilage at the ends of the bone

d. *a* and *b*

e. *a*, *b*, and *c*

____ 4. In a long bone,

a. the shaft is called the diaphysis

b. red marrow is the site of blood cell production

c. chondroblasts produce the bone cells

d. *a* and *b*

e. *a*, *b*, and *c*

____ 5. Of the following connective tissue types, which is found on the articulating surfaces of long bones?

a. elastic cartilage

b. hyaline cartilage

c. reticular tissue

d. dense irregular collagenous tissue

____ 6. Of the following pairs of articulations, which pair is *not* correctly matched?

a. symphysis and bodies of adjacent vertebrae

b. synchondrosis and ulna and radius

c. syndesmosis and the two coxae

d. synovial and costochondral joints

____ 7. A muscle fiber is a single cell consisting of all but which of the following components?

a. sarcolemma

b. sarcoplasm

    c. cilia

    d. myofibrils

___ 8. Which of the following best describes myosin molecules?

    a. They consist of double helix structures.

    b. The proteins F-myosin and G-myosin make up the myosin molecule.

    c. They consist of two globular heads and a rod-like portion.

    d. They consist of A bands and I bands.

___ 9. What is the term for the outermost layer of connective tissue on the skeletal muscle?

    a. epimysium

    b. sarcomysium

    c. endomysium

    d. perimysium

___ 10. What major characteristic distinguishes connective tissue from other tissue?

    a. mechanism of secretion

    b. extracellular matrix

    c. important function in diffusion

    d. ability to conduct electrical impulses

___ 11. Of the following connective tissue types, which is found within the lymph nodes, spleen, and bone marrow?

    a. elastic cartilage

    b. hyaline cartilage

    c. reticular tissue

    d. dense irregular collagenous tissue

___ 12. What makes up the extracellular matrix of cartilage?

    a. protein filaments and proteoglycan aggregates

    b. minerals

    c. fluid

    d. dense connective tissue

___ 13. Which of the following is *not* considered connective tissue?

    a. blood

    b. stratified epithelium

    c. bone

    d. adipose tissue

___ 14. Where are the SA node and the AV node located?

    a. the right atrium

    b. the right ventricle

    c. the right atrium and right ventricle, respectively

    d. the left atrium

___ 15. Of the following statements, which is *not* true of cardiac muscle cells?

    a. Cardiac muscle cells are similar in design to skeletal muscle cells.

    b. Cardiac muscle cells are joined by intercalated discs.

    c. Cardiac muscle cells are well supplied with blood vessels.

    d. Cardiac muscle cells contain a well-developed T-tubule system.

___ 16. Which of the following is a true statement about the heart?

    a. It contains a fibrous pericardium that holds it in place.

    b. It is composed of two ventricles separated by an interatrial septum.

    c. It has an endomysium, perimysium, and epimysium forming its wall.

    d. It is supplied by coronary arteries branching off the right and left subclavian arteries.

___ 17. Which of the following is true regarding the external anatomy of the heart?

    a. Each atrium has a flap of tissue called an auricle.

    b. The aorta exits the right ventricle.

    c. The four pulmonary veins enter the right atrium.

    d. The pulmonary trunk exits the left ventricle.

___ 18. Deoxygenated blood returning from the body enters the superior and inferior venae cavae. What is the correct sequence of events for blood flow through the heart?

    a. right atrium, right ventricle, pulmonary arteries, tricuspid valve

    b. right atrium, tricuspid valve, right ventricle, pulmonary veins

    c. right atrium, tricuspid valve, right ventricle, pulmonary arteries

    d. right atrium, mitral valve, right ventricle, pulmonary veins

___ 19. Which of the following is true of coronary circulation?

    a. A large coronary sinus separates the right and left ventricles.

    b. The left coronary artery and the right anterior interventricular artery arise from the sinus of Valsalva.

    c. The right circumflex artery eventually anastomoses with the circumflex artery.

    d. The right coronary artery gives rise to the circumflex arteries.

___ 20. Which of the following are correct regarding aging and the heart?

    a. Hypertrophy of the left ventricle is common.

    b. Maximum heart rate decreases.

    c. Heart valves may function abnormally.

    d. *a* and *b*

    e. *a*, *b*, and *c*

___ 21. The heart wall contains

    a. an outer epicardium

    b. a middle layer responsible for contraction

    c. an endocardium to reduce friction

    d. *a* and *b*

    e. *a*, *b*, and *c*

___ 22. The trachea extends from which of the following?

    a. larynx to pharynx

    b. nose to pharynx

    c. pharynx to primary bronchi

    d. larynx to primary bronchi

___ 23. Anatomically, the respiratory system is divided into which of the following?

    a. superior meatus, middle meatus, and inferior meatus

    b. pharynx, olfactory epithelium, and cricoid cartilage

    c. conducting zone structures and paranasal sinuses

    d. upper respiratory tract and lower respiratory tract

___ 24. Which of the following is an accurate statement about the larynx?

    a. It is an organ of both the respiratory and digestive systems located at the back of the oral and nasal cavities.

    b. It helps to filter air.

    c. It contains nine cartilages and vocal folds.

    d. It is located between the phalanx and pharynx.

___ 25. How many lobes does the right lung have?

    a. one

    b. two

    c. three

    d. four

___ 26. Along with the ribs and costal cartilages, what is (are) contained in the thoracic cage?

    a. diaphragm

    b. sternum and diaphragm

    c. sternum and intercostals

    d. sternum and vertebrae

___ 27. Which of the following statements is true of the vertebral column?

    a. Each thoracic vertebra contains a peg-like projection called the dens, or odontoid process, for articulation with the ribs.

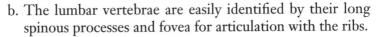

b. The lumbar vertebrae are easily identified by their long spinous processes and fovea for articulation with the ribs.

c. The 12 thoracic vertebrae have transverse foramina and long, downward spinous processes.

d. The seven cervical vertebrae have transverse foramina.

___ 28. Which of the following is true of the appendicular skeleton?

a. It consists of upper and lower limbs and the girdles that attach to the limbs.

b. It consists of the skull, vertebrae, thoracic cage, and shoulder girdle.

c. It consists of the bones that form the axis of the body.

d. It supports and protects the organs of the head, neck, and trunk.

___ 29. Which of the following is true of the major bones of the body?

a. The mandible and maxilla possess alveolar processes with sockets for the attachment ossicles of the middle ear.

b. Eight tarsal bones make up the ankle.

c. The occipital bone forms the lower sides of the cranium and contains a mastoid process that is easily palpated behind the earlobe.

d. The femur articulates with the head of the coxa, the medial and lateral condyles of the tibia, and the patella.

___ 30. Which of the following best describes the trapezius?

a. It inserts at the clavicle, acromion process, and scapular spine and elevates, depresses, retracts, and fixes the scapula.

b. It is innervated by the subclavian nerve and elevates, depresses, retracts, and fixes the scapula.

c. It originates at the first to the ninth ribs and adducts and abducts the upper arm.

d. It inserts at the sternum, clavicle, and acromion process and adducts and abducts the upper arm.

___ 31. Of the following, which is (are) true about the pectoralis major?

a. It adducts, flexes, and medially rotates the arm.

b. It inserts on the greater tubercle of the humerus.

c. It is innervated by the axillary nerve.

d. *a* and *b* only

e. *a*, *b*, and *c*

___ 32. Compression of the abdomen is accomplished by the external obliques and which of the following muscles?

    a. pectoralis major, rectus abdominis, and transverse abdominis

    b. rectus abdominis, internal abdominal obliques, and transverse abdominis

    c. rectus abdominis, diaphragm, and internal abdominal obliques

    d. transverse abdominis, internal abdominal obliques, and diaphragm

___ 33. Which of the following is (are) true of the erector spinae muscles?

    a. They originate as a large fleshy mass in the sacral area of the back.

    b. They consist of the iliocostalis, longissimus, and the spinalis muscles.

    c. They extend the vertebral column and flex the hip.

    d. *a* and *b* only

    e. *a*, *b*, and *c*

___ 34. Which of the following is (are) true about the gluteus maximus?

    a. It contributes most of the mass of the buttocks.

    b. It abducts and laterally rotates the thigh.

    c. It flexes the thigh.

    d. *a* and *b* only

    e. *a*, *b*, and *c*

___ 35. Which muscles are involved in thigh extension?

    a. the gluteus medius

    b. the hamstrings

    c. the semitendinosus, biceps femoris, and the semimembranosus

d. *a* and *b* only

e. *a*, *b*, and *c*

____ 36. Which movements are associated with the gastrocnemius?

  a. extending the four lateral toes and flexing the leg

  b. plantar flexion of the foot and flexing the leg

  c. extending the four lateral toes and extending the great toe

  d. plantar flexion of the foot and extending the great toe

____ 37. When the arm is flexed to a 90° position and movement is in the transverse plane, it is termed

  a. horizontal abduction

  b. horizontal adduction

  c. pronation

  d. left and right rotation

____ 38. From the anatomical position, what are the two primary movements occurring in the sagittal plane in addition to flexion?

  a. extension and rotation

  b. extension and hyperextension

  c. extension and adduction

  d. extension and hyperflexion

____ 39. What movement returns a body segment to the anatomical position?

  a. flexion

  b. extension

  c. inversion

  d. eversion

____ 40. What action moves a body segment away from the midline of the body?

  a. flexion

  b. extension

  c. abduction

  d. adduction

___ 41. What movements occur within the frontal plane?
    a. flexion, extension, rotation
    b. flexion, abduction, adduction
    c. inversion, abduction, adduction
    d. medial and lateral rotation

___ 42. What name is given to movement beyond the anatomical position when starting from a position of extension?
    a. abduction
    b. extension
    c. hyperflexion
    d. hyperextension

___ 43. The movement of which parts of the body is described by left and right rotation?
    a. thigh, leg, and foot
    b. head, neck, and trunk
    c. head and neck
    d. trunk, hip, and foot

___ 44. An example of what movement(s) is produced by the circular movement of a limb?
    a. circumcision
    b. circumduction
    c. circumflexion
    d. circumvention
    e. *a* and *b* only

___ 45. When a muscle contracts and causes movement of a segment at a joint, it is acting
    a. as an antagonist
    b. as an unstabilizer
    c. as an agonist
    d. as a stabilizer

___ 46. Some muscles act to eliminate unwanted movement by an agonist. This is termed

a. active insufficiency

b. passive insufficiency

c. stabilizer

d. neutralizer

___ 47. Which of the following is a true statement about fibrous joints?

a. They have no joint cavity and include sutures and syndesmoses.

b. They have no joint cavity and include bursae and synchondroses.

c. They are incapable of any movement.

d. They contain hyaline cartilage between bone segments.

___ 48. Which of the following is a true statement about cartilaginous joints?

a. They are freely movable.

b. They contain a synovial membrane.

c. They could be identified with the symphysis pubis.

d. They include sutures, gomphoses, and syndesmoses.

___ 49. Which of the following best describes synovial joints?

a. They are slightly movable and have articular cartilage on the ends of the bone.

b. They are slightly movable and include symphyses.

c. They have articular cartilage on the ends of the bones and a synovial membrane that produces synovial fluid.

d. They include symphyses and have a synovial membrane that produces synovial fluid.

___ 50. Which of the following statements is true of stability?

a. The smaller the base of support, the more stable the body.

b. Movement toward the midline of the body in one direction will cause the center of gravity to shift away from that direction, making the body more stable.

c. A foot position that allows for a small base of support in the direction of the movement will provide added stability.

d. Stability is directly proportional to the distance of the line of gravity from the limits of the base of support.

____ 51. What is an individual's ability to control equilibrium called?

    a. stability

    b. balance

    c. static motion

    d. torque

____ 52. When is the body's ability to maintain equilibrium enhanced?

    a. when opposing forces acting on the body are not equal

    b. when the center of gravity is vertically positioned near the edge of the base of support

    c. when body mass is increased and the base of support is directed in the line of action of the external force

    d. when the friction between the body and the surface area is decreased

____ 53. Which of the following paired terms indicate abnormal back curvatures commonly called "hunched back" and "hollow back," respectively?

    a. lordosis–kyphosis

    b. kyphosis–lordosis

    c. scoliosis–lordosis

    d. lordosis–scoliosis

____ 54. What is scoliosis?

    a. a lateral deviation of the spine

    b. an anterior exaggeration of the lumbar curve

    c. exaggerated posterior thoracic convexity

    d. exaggerated posterior lumbar concavity

____ 55. What protocols are included in training programs designed to improve strength?

    a. isometric

    b. isotonic with constant or varying resistance

    c. isokinetic

    d. all of these

____ 56. What name is given to an exercise designed to develop strength that puts a muscle group on stretch prior to its contraction?

a. repetitions maximum

b. isokinetic

c. plyometric

d. progressive resistive

___ 57. For optimal strength gains, a typical weight-training program would include which of the following?

a. one set of biceps curls with 10-pound weights, one day a week, for 10 weeks

b. multiple exercises, training 2-3 times per week, performing between 3RM and 12RM

c. one set of exercises with 20RM protocol

d. Lift one time per week.

e. Adhere to the overload principle.

___ 58. Which of the following approaches is (are) recommended to improve flexibility?

a. Minimize the effect of muscle spindles and maximize the effect of golgi tendon organs.

b. Employ a technique called static stretching.

c. Employ a technique called reciprocal inhibition.

d. *a* and *b*

e. *a*, *b*, and *c*

___ 59. One of the most effective stretching procedures is termed

a. passive stretching

b. active stretching

c. proprioceptive neuromuscular facilitation

d. *a* and *b*

e. *a*, *b*, and *c*

___ 60. The risk of injury increases when joint flexibility is

a. extremely low

b. extremely high

c. imbalanced between dominant and nondominant sides of the body

d. *a* and *b*

e. *a*, *b*, and *c*

___ 61. Match the type of joint and corresponding movement associated with the shoulder.

    a. gliding–hyperextension

    b. pivot–pronation

    c. ball and socket–circumduction

    d. hinge–flexion

___ 62. Which of the following describes the type of joint in which the articulating surfaces are nearly flat and where the only movement allowed is a monoaxial motion confined to one plane?

    a. pivot

    b. gliding

    c. condyloid

    d. ball and socket

___ 63. Choose the correctly matched type of joint and corresponding movement, and example.

    a. plane–monoaxial; processes between vertebrae

    b. saddle–circumduction; knee

    c. ellipsoid–flexion; shoulder

    d. pivot–biaxial rotation; elbow

___ 64. Where might you find a joint that has one convex articulating bone surface and one concave articulating bone surface with movement restricted to a hinge-like motion?

    a. knee

    b. neck

    c. shoulder

    d. hip

___ 65. The ankle joint

    a. is a special hinge joint

    b. involves the tibia, fibula, and talus

    c. is a complex ellipsoid joint

    d. *a* and *b*

    e. *a*, *b*, and *c*

___ 66. What movements are included in frontal plane movements of the hip?

    a. lateral flexion and adduction

    b. adduction and abduction

    c. lateral flexion and lateral extension

    d. adduction and lateral extension

___ 67. What movements are included in the transverse plane movements of the forearm?

    a. outward and inward rotation

    b. pronation and supination

    c. elevation and depression

    d. eversion and inversion

    e. lateral flexion

___ 68. The degree of movement within a specific joint (ROM) is limited by which of the following?

    a. bony structures of two articulating surfaces

    b. length of the ligaments

    c. elasticity of the connective tissues

    d. *a* and *b*

    e. *a*, *b*, and *c*

___ 69. What is the term for the fluid force that enables flotation?

    a. drag

    b. lift

    c. buoyancy

    d. Magnus effect

___ 70. What is the term for the fluid force that acts to slow a cyclist moving through that fluid?

    a. turbulence

    b. drag

    c. lift

    d. friction

___ 71. Propulsion in swimming results from a complex interplay of what two fluid forces?

    a. Magnus effect and drag

    b. skin friction and wave drag

    c. propulsive lift and loft

    d. propulsive lift and propulsive drag

___ 72. Which of the following biomechanical principles are applicable when one lifts a heavy object?

    a. establishing a base of support as close as possible to the load being carried and lowering the body into position by flexing the knees, hips, and ankles

    b. stabilizing the vertebral column in the flexed position and lowering the body into position by flexing at the waist

    c. stabilizing the vertebral column in the flexed position and raising the load with the extensor muscles of the legs

    d. establishing a base of support as far as possible from the load being carried and lowering the body into position by flexing the knees, hips, and ankles

___ 73. Rapidly executing a lift

    a. increases intra-abdominal pressure

    b. increases compression and shear forces on the spine

    c. increases load on the third lumbar disc, especially in the supine position

    d. results in the flexion relaxation phenomenon

___ 74. Forward speed during walking and running results from what two elements?

    a. vertical force and time of ground contact

    b. stride length and stride frequency

    c. stride frequency and vertical push

    d. stride length and horizontal lift

___ 75. During walking, the foot applies a force to the ground and there follows an equal and opposite ground reaction force to the foot. This is an example of which of Newton's laws of motion?

a. first

b. second

c. third

d. fourth

___ 76. A cyclist wears a streamlined helmet

a. to reduce drag

b. to reduce turbulence created by the trailing edge

c. to minimize metabolic cost during the ride

d. *a* and *b*

e. *a*, *b*, and *c*

___ 77. Which statement correctly identifies the measurement site for abdominal circumference?

a. midway between the xiphoid process and the umbilicus

b. on the natural fold of the iliac crest

c. at the level of the umbilicus

d. at the narrowest part of the torso above the umbilicus

___ 78. What is the correct anatomic landmark site for determining peripheral pulse?

a. femoral pulse—anterior thigh, posterior to the inguinal ligament, midway between the anterior superior iliac spine and the pubis symphysis

b. popliteal—deep within the patellar fossa

c. radial pulse—distal end of the ulna

d. *a* and *b*

e. *a*, *b*, and *c*

___ 79. When taking a carotid pulse,

a. press two fingers in the groove formed by the larynx and the sternocleidomastoid muscles

b. if one presses too hard, a baroreceptor response will be elicited

c. fainting might result in extreme cases

d. *a* and *b*

e. *a*, *b*, and *c*

___ 80. Which of the following is the correct placement of cuff and bladder during blood pressure assessment?

    a. Lower edge of the cuff is placed one inch above the antecubital space on the frontal aspect of the elbow.

    b. Always place the cuff on the right arm.

    c. Lower edge of cuff is placed one inch below the midaxillary line.

    d. *a* and *b*

    e. *a, b,* and *c*

___ 81. During blood pressure measurement, the stethoscope head should be placed

    a. one inch above the antecubital space on the exterior aspect of the elbow

    b. popliteal space on the frontal aspect of the elbow

    c. medial antecubital space

    d. *a* and *b*

    e. *a, b,* and *c*

___ 82. Which of the following landmarks are correct for skinfold assessment?

    a. waist—narrowest part of the torso

    b. waist—above the umbilicus and below the xiphoid process

    c. waist—gluteal fold

    d. *a* and *b*

    e. *a, b,* and *c*

___ 83. Which of the following landmarks are correct for skinfold assessment?

    a. suprailiac—diagonal fold in line with the natural angle of the iliac crest

    b. subscapular—45° angle one to two cm below the inferior angle of the scapula

    c. abdominal—vertical fold 23 cm to the right of the umbilicus

    d. *a* and *b*

    e. *a, b,* and *c*

___ 84. The ratio of waist to hip (WHR) circumferences
   a. reflects central versus peripheral fat pattern
   b. is an index of upper- versus lower-body fat distribution
   c. can be used to estimate body composition
   d. *a* and *b*
   e. *a, b,* and *c*

___ 85. Exercise has many beneficial effects on the health of the heart. Which of the following are true for heart health and exercise?
   a. Hypertrophy occurs from a gradual increase in pressure in the aorta.
   b. Myocardial cells accumulate lipid and collagen fibers to increase cardiac tissue.
   c. Improved functional capacity providing no conditions develop that cause the increase in workload to be harmful to the heart.
   d. *a* and *b*
   e. *a, b,* and *c*

___ 86. Exercise during pregnancy
   a. is encouraged
   b. is beneficial to women and helps them recover more quickly after delivery
   c. is counterproductive to stable metabolism of the fetus
   d. *a* and *b*
   e. *a, b,* and *c*

___ 87. Treatments for osteoporosis
   a. are designed to reduce bone loss or increase bone formation
   b. include an increase in calcium and vitamin D to the diet
   c. include exercise, such as walking or using light weights
   d. *a* and *b*
   e. *a, b,* and *c*

___ 88. The optimal window of loading during exercise for a healthy individual includes consideration of

a. magnitude of the force

b. rate at which the force is applied

c. load repetition

d. *a* and *b*

e. *a, b,* and *c*

___ 89. Loading the human body during exercise

a. alters the size, shape, and structure of bone

b. can increase cancellous and cortical bone

c. increases bone dimensions during microgravity

d. *a* and *b*

e. *a, b,* and *c*

___ 90. Which of the following muscle actions and associated plane of action is (are) correct?

a. flexion—sagittal plane

b. abduction—transverse plane

c. plantar flexion—frontal plane

d. *a* and *b*

e. *a, b,* and *c*

___ 91. Improper spinal alignment during activity can result in

a. low back pain

b. lumbar strain

c. lumbar sprain

d. *a* and *b*

e. *a, b,* and *c*

___ 92. The myotatic reflex

a. provokes reflex contraction in a stretched muscle

b. inhibits tension development in antagonist muscles

c. results in immediate development of muscle tension

d. *a* and *b*

e. *a, b,* and *c*

REFERENCES FOR FURTHER STUDY

1. ACSM. (2001). *ACSM's resource manual for guidelines for exercise testing and prescription* (4th ed.). Philadelphia: Lippincott Williams & Wilkins.
2. Hall, S.J. (2003). *Basic biomechanics* (4th ed.). Boston: McGraw-Hill.
3. McArdle, W.D., Katch, F.I., & Katch, V.I. (2001). *Exercise physiology: Energy, nutrition, and human performance* (5th ed.). Baltimore: Williams & Wilkins.
4. Seeley, R.R., Stephens, T.D., & Tate, P. (2003). *Anatomy and physiology* (6th ed.). Boston: McGraw-Hill.

ANSWERS

Question number	Answer	KSA number	Reference	Page number
1	d	1.1.0.1	4	168
2	a	1.1.0.1	4	179
3	e	1.1.0.1	4	176-178
4	d	1.1.0.1	4	168
5	b	1.1.0.1	4	124
6	a	1.1.0.1	4	242
7	c	1.1.0.1	4	275
8	c	1.1.0.1	4	276
9	a	1.1.0.1	4	274
10	b	1.1.0.1	4	118
11	c	1.1.0.1	4	124
12	a	1.1.0.1	4	118
13	b	1.1.0.1	4	119
14	a	1.1.0.2	4	680
15	d	1.1.0.2	4	679
16	a	1.1.0.2	4	670

Question number	Answer	KSA number	Reference	Page number
17	a	1.1.0.2	4	672
18	c	1.1.0.2	4	678
19	c	1.1.0.2	4	672
20	e	1.1.0.2	4	699
21	e	1.1.0.2	4	670
22	d	1.1.0.2	4	817
23	d	1.1.0.2	4	814
24	c	1.1.0.2	4	816
25	c	1.1.0.2	4	821
26	d	1.1.0.3	4	225
27	d	1.1.0.3	4	217
28	a	1.1.0.3	4	225
29	d	1.1.0.3	4	201, 215, 233, 235
30	a	1.1.0.3	4	338
31	d	1.1.0.3	4	340
32	b	1.1.0.3	4	334
33	d	1.1.0.3	4	332
34	d	1.1.0.3	4	349
35	e	1.1.0.3	4	352
36	b	1.1.0.3	4	354
37	a	1.1.0.4	2	39
38	b	1.1.0.4	2	35
39	b	1.1.0.4	2	35
40	c	1.1.0.4	2	36

Question number	Answer	KSA number	Reference	Page number
41	c	1.1.0.4	2	36
42	d	1.1.0.4	2	35
43	b	1.1.0.4	2	38
44	b	1.1.0.4	2	40
45	c	1.1.0.5	2	159
46	d	1.1.0.5	2	160
47	a	1.1.0.5	2	118
48	c	1.1.0.5	2	118
49	c	1.1.0.5	2	119
50	d	1.1.1.2	2	441
51	b	1.1.1.2	2	441
52	c	1.1.1.2	2	444-445
53	b	1.1.1.3	2	284
54	a	1.1.1.3	2	284
55	d	1.1.1.4	3	510
56	c	1.1.1.4	3	524
57	b	1.1.1.4	3	511
58	e	1.1.1.5	2	130, 132
59	c	1.1.1.5	2	132
60	e	1.1.1.5	2	128
61	c	2.1.0.1	4	247
62	b	2.1.0.1	4	247
63	a	2.1.0.1	4	247
64	a	2.1.0.1	4	248

Question number	Answer	KSA number	Reference	Page number
65	d	2.1.0.1	4	262
66	b	2.1.0.1	2	36
67	b	2.1.0.1	2	39
68	e	2.1.0.1	2	126
69	c	2.1.1	2	483
70	b	2.1.1	2	486
71	d	2.1.1	2	500
72	a	2.1.1	2	299
73	b	2.1.1	2	298
74	b	2.1.1	1	117
75	c	2.1.1	1	108
76	d	2.1.1	2	490
77	c	2.1.0.4	1	101
78	a	2.1.0.2	1	97
79	e	2.1.0.2	1	97
80	a	2.1.0.3	1	96
81	c	2.1.0.3	1	96
82	d	2.1.0.4	1	103
83	e	2.1.0.4	1	99
84	b	2.1.0.4	1	393
85	c	1.1.0	4	699
86	d	1.1.0	4	1083
87	e	1.1.0	4	190
88	e	1.1.0	1	110

Question number	Answer	KSA number	Reference	Page number
89	d	1.1.1	1	111
90	a	1.1.1.1	2	35
91	e	1.1.1.2	1	496
92	c	1.1.1.6	2	130

Exercise Physiology

The ACSM KSA category of Exercise Physiology contains 35 objectives. In the Health/Fitness Instructor certification examination you are likely to encounter approximately 20 questions from this KSA category.

PRACTICE QUESTIONS

Instructions: Each question is followed by either four or five possible answers. Select the *best* answer to the question.

_____ 1. What is true about a metabolic process requiring no O_2?

    a. It is termed *aerobic* and could be written as ATP + H_2O ← ADP + Pi + Energy.

    b. It is termed *anaerobic* and could be written as ATP + H_2O ← ADP + Pi + Energy.

    c. It is found exclusively in the mitochondria of a cell.

    d. It is termed *Krebs cycle*; it could be written as CP + ADP ← ATP + C + Energy.

_____ 2. Which of the following statements is (are) true regarding aerobic metabolism?

    a. It requires O_2 and involves a mitochondrial process in which inorganic phosphate is coupled to ADP via the electron transport chain.

    b. It can utilize muscle glycogen, blood glucose, plasma-free fatty acids, and intramuscular fats.

    c. It is useful for long-term activities and is the term commonly used to describe the level of O_2 consumption at which there is a rapid rise in blood lactate.

    d. *a* and *b*

____ 3. Generally, what contributes most to intense activity and long-lasting activity, respectively?

    a. anaerobic sources; aerobic sources

    b. oxidation of fat; metabolism of glucose

    c. aerobic sources; anaerobic sources

    d. oxidation of glucose; the ATP-PC system

____ 4. Which of the following is (are) true about short-term, high-intensity exercise?

    a. Aerobic metabolism provides the primary source of ATP.

    b. A half-mile swim and the 1,500-meter run are good examples.

    c. It typically lasts 5 to 60 seconds, and the ATP-PC system and anaerobic glycolysis are preferentially used to provide ATP.

    d. *b* and *c*

____ 5. What term refers to the volume of blood pumped through the aorta every minute?

    a. stroke volume

    b. ejection fraction

    c. end-systolic volume

    d. cardiac output

____ 6. What term refers to the body's ability to transport and utilize O_2 during rest or exercise?

    a. the respiratory exchange ratio

    b. $\dot{V}O_2$

    c. $\dot{V}O_2$max

    d. pulmonary ventilation

___ 7. Which of the following is true regarding hyperventilation?

    a. It is increased pulmonary ventilation with a retention of carbon dioxide.

    b. It is due to an increase in expiration of air.

    c. It occurs at approximately 40 percent $\dot{V}O_2max$.

    d. It can lead to respiratory alkalosis without physiological compensation.

___ 8. What term refers to the highest arterial BP recorded during the cardiac cycle?

    a. SBP

    b. DBP

    c. mean arterial BP

    d. total peripheral resistance

___ 9. What is the pressure in the arterial system when the cardiac muscle is relaxed, and what is the normal value?

    a. SBP; typically 120 mmHg

    b. DBP; typically 80 mmHg

    c. mean arterial pressure; typically 90 mmHg

    d. total peripheral resistance; typically 100 mmHg

___ 10. What is true about myocardial ischemia?

    a. It is a condition of inadequate blood flow.

    b. It may be accompanied by atherosclerosis.

    c. It may have concomitant angina pectoris.

    d. *a* and *b*

    e. *a*, *b*, and *c*

___ 11. What is true about tachycardia?

    a. It is exemplified by a HR greater than 100 beats per minute.

    b. It is a response to fever, nervous excitement, or exercise.

    c. It acts to increase the O_2 delivered to the cells of the body via an increase in circulation.

    d. *a* and *b*

    e. *a*, *b*, and *c*

_____ 12. Which is true about bradycardia?

    a. It is defined as a condition in which the HR is less than 60 beats per minute.

    b. It is a condition that occurs during sleep and is seen in some physically fit people.

    c. It is also called sick sinus syndrome.

    d. *a* and *b*

    e. *a*, *b*, and *c*

_____ 13. What is true about myocardial infarction?

    a. It is also called heart attack.

    b. It is death of a portion of the heart muscle.

    c. It is caused by obstruction in a coronary artery due to atherosclerosis or embolism.

    d. *a* and *b*

    e. *a*, *b*, and *c*

_____ 14. What is true about angina pectoris?

    a. It is a sudden pain in the chest area, most often due to a lack of O_2 to the heart tissue.

    b. It is a painless episode of coronary insufficiency.

    c. It is a tumor of the heart muscle.

    d. It occurs quite often during exercise.

    e. It is a thin, triangular muscle of the upper chest wall beneath the pectoralis major.

_____ 15. In general, what nutrient combination is used preferentially during high-intensity activity and metabolized preferentially during long-term activity, respectively?

    a. CHO, FAT

    b. FAT, CHO

    c. FAT, PRO

    d. PRO, FAT

_____ 16. Which of the following exercise prescriptions meet the recommended cardiorespiratory fitness guidelines?

a. intensity = 40/50 to 85 percent $\dot{V}O_2R$; frequency = three times per week; duration = time required to expend 200 kcal

b. intensity = 40/50 percent HRR; frequency = three times per week; duration = 200 kcal per session

c. intensity = 55/60 to 90 percent HR max; frequency = three times per week; duration = 30 minutes per session

d. *a* and *b*

e. *a*, *b*, and *c*

___ 17. An optimal program for strength training would include which of the following guidelines?

a. a minimum of 8 to 10 different exercises involving the major muscle groups

b. exercises that involve the full ROM

c. performance at an intensity level that would cause fatigue within 8 to 12 repetitions

d. *a*, *b*, and *c*

___ 18. Which of the following describes the best training to improve flexibility?

a. static stretching; a minimum of two to three days per week; holding each stretch to position of mild discomfort

b. ballistic stretching; five sessions per week; holding each stretch for one to two seconds

c. static stretching; two sessions per week; holding each stretch for 10 to 60 seconds (depending upon flexibility training level)

d. a combination of static and ballistic stretching (dependent upon joint area); two sessions per week; repeating each stretch 10 times with no limit on stretch holding time

___ 19. There is a great concern about body fat and its association with obesity and health-related problems. Which of the following statements identifies a component of fitness as it relates to body fat?

a. Recommended body fat percentages for men over the age of 56 years should be between 10 and 25 percent.

b. Recommended body fat percentages for athletic women should be between 12 and 22 percent.

c. A BMI of below 25 kg/m^2 is desirable.

d. *a* and *b*

e. *a, b,* and *c*

___ 20. What are the two most common sites for pulse palpation of HR during exercise?

a. brachial artery and carotid artery

b. radial artery and temporal artery

c. femoral artery and radial artery

d. carotid artery and temporal artery

e. femoral artery and carotid artery

___ 21. Premature ventricular contractions (PVCs)

a. occur when a site in the ventricle fires before the next depolarization from the SA node

b. are indicative of cardiac disease

c. are recognized by the absence of a QRS complex

d. *a* and *b*

e. *a, b,* and *c*

___ 22. During an acute bout of aerobic exercise, which of the following occur(s)?

a. BP increases linearly with exercise intensity.

b. HR increases linearly with exercise intensity.

c. SV increases linearly with exercise intensity.

d. *a* and *b*

e. *a, b,* and *c*

___ 23. Which of the following accurately describe(s) O$_2$ consumption?

a. It increases linearly until a steady state is reached in a single bout of exercise.

b. It increases linearly during graded exercise.

c. It increases linearly over time during a steady state exercise bout.

d. *a* and *b*

e. *a*, *b*, and *c*

_____ 24. Which of the following occur(s) during an isometric grip strength test?

a. SBP increases with a concomitant decrease in DBP.

b. HR increases linearly until a steady state is reached.

c. HR and DBP increase over time.

d. *a* and *b*

e. *a*, *b*, and *c*

_____ 25. Which of the following occur(s) when a static contraction is performed at 60 percent MVC?

a. Blood flow to the muscle is reduced.

b. SBP may exceed 200 mmHg.

c. HR increases moderately.

d. *a* and *b*

e. *a*, *b*, and *c*

_____ 26. What causes elevated O_2 levels observed during postexercise?

a. the replenishment of PC in the muscle and O_2 in the blood and tissues

b. an elevated HR and BP

c. physiological consequences as a result of elevated body temperature

d. *a* and *b*

e. *a*, *b*, and *c*

_____ 27. What result would be expected for a given bout of exercise after a person engages in endurance training?

a. an improved SV

b. a lower HR

c. an increased Q

d. *a* and *b*

e. *a*, *b*, and *c*

___ 28. Jay and Lynn began an exercise program together. They jogged at 75 percent of their $\dot{V}O_2$max, four times a week, for 30 minutes per session. After two months, they wondered what physiological changes may have occurred as a result of their training. Please note that Jay is 6 feet 1 inches and 180 pounds; Lynn is 5 feet 2 inches and 115 pounds. What cardiovascular changes would be expected after completion of their training program?

    a. Lynn's $\dot{V}O_2$max will be lower than Jay's $\dot{V}O_2$max.

    b. Jay's and Lynn's $\dot{V}O_2$max will be equal.

    c. Jay's BP will be increased at rest.

    d. Lynn's BP will be increased at rest.

___ 29. The resting and submaximal bradycardic response to training is due to

    a. decreased intrinsic firing rate at the SA node

    b. increased parasympathetic tone

    c. small decrease in sympathetic tone

    d. *a* and *b*

    e. *a*, *b*, and *c*

___ 30. What physiological adaptation(s) occur(s) as a result of strength training?

    a. an increase in muscle mass

    b. hypertrophy

    c. hyperplasia

    d. *a* and *b*

    e. *a*, *b*, and *c*

___ 31. What central nervous system adaptation(s) result(s) from a strength-training program?

    a. an increase in the number of motor units recruited

    b. a modification in the firing rates of motor units

    c. an enhancement in motor unit synchronization during a movement pattern

    d. a removal of neural inhibition

    e. all of these

___ 32. To what can we attribute the gains in strength that occur early (first three weeks) in a strength-training program?

    a. an enlargement of the muscle

    b. hyperplasia

    c. hypertrophy

    d. neural adaptation

    e. all of these

___ 33. After a six-month progressive resistive-exercise strength-training program, which of the following will be noted in females when compared to male counterparts?

    a. similar gains in relative strength

    b. less hypertrophy

    c. more atrophy

    d. *a* and *b*

    e. *a*, *b*, and *c*

___ 34. According to research conducted thus far on resistance training, what are some of the early increases in voluntary strength attributable to?

    a. improved coordination

    b. psychologic disinhibition

    c. increased activation of the prime mover muscles

    d. *a* and *b*

    e. *a*, *b*, and *c*

___ 35. What occurs in the early stages of strength training?

    a. Muscle strength increases more than muscle size.

    b. Muscle size increases more than muscle strength.

    c. There is an increase in oxidative enzyme activities within the muscle.

    d. HR responses to work show little change.

___ 36. What would be expected in a strength-training program conducted for six weeks?

    a. gains in strength due to muscle hypertrophy

    b. gains in strength due to neural adaptations

    c. an increase in the number of type IIa fibers

    d. *a* and *b*

    e. *a*, *b*, and *c*

___ 37. Which of the following should be monitored to assess the appropriate level of exercise intensity during a GXT?

    a. rating of perceived exertion

    b. heart rate

    c. profuse sweating

    d. *a* and *b*

    e. *a*, *b*, and *c*

___ 38. Which of the following is (are) true about warm-up activities before exercise?

    a. They prepare the body for vigorous activity.

    b. They may prevent injury.

    c. They allow the body to redirect blood to the muscles.

    d. They may induce faster muscle contraction and relaxation.

    e. All of these are true.

___ 39. Optimal warm-up before activity results in which of the following?

    a. less muscle resistance when the warm-up is performed similarly to the activity (e.g., a baseball pitcher practicing at 50 percent of normal effort)

    b. facilitated nerve transmission and motor unit recruitment

    c. facilitated oxygen delivery and use by the muscle

    d. *a* and *b*

    e. *a*, *b*, and *c*

___ 40. What is (are) the primary physiological benefit(s) to be gained during a cool-down after exercise?

    a. promotes a quicker return of HR and BP to normal values

    b. stimulates the return of pooled blood from limbs to the central circulation

c. facilitates lactate removal

d. *a* and *b*

e. *a*, *b*, and *c*

___ 41. The benefits of warm-up and cool-down include all but which of the following?

   a. an increased breakdown of oxyhemoglobin to enhance O_2 delivery to the muscle

   b. an inhibition of catecholamine release, perhaps preventing arrhythmias

   c. a reduction in the occurrence of myocardial infarction

   d. a reduction in the viscosity of muscle, thereby improving mechanical efficiency and power

   e. a psychological preparation for the activity

___ 42. Which of the following is (are) true regarding an active cool-down period following exercise?

   a. It enhances removal of metabolic waste from the blood, which in susceptible individuals may prevent a cardiac arrhythmia.

   b. It prevents blood pooling in the legs and thereby may prevent delayed muscle stiffening.

   c. Older individuals benefit from long periods of cool-down.

   d. *a* and *b*

   e. *a*, *b*, and *c*

___ 43. Why do exercise and training become more difficult as one ascends to higher altitudes?

   a. The partial pressure of O_2 decreases at increased altitudes with a concomitant decrease in O_2 saturation.

   b. $\dot{V}O_2$max decreases at increased altitudes.

   c. Respiratory alkalosis develops shortly after arrival at increased altitudes.

   d. *a* and *b*

   e. *a*, *b*, and *c*

___ 44. Which of the following pairs of conditions would be true during exercise at increased altitudes?

    a. decrease in barometric pressure; reduction of O_2 saturation

    b. submaximal workload; higher HR

    c. training at altitude; carryover in training effect at sea level

    d. *a* and *b*

    e. *a*, *b*, and *c*

___ 45. Hyperventilation

    a. refers to an increase in pulmonary ventilation

    b. provides more oxygen than needed

    c. increases plasma pH

    d. *a* and *b*

    e. *a*, *b*, and *c*

___ 46. Dyspnea

    a. refers to an inordinate shortness of breath

    b. results in elevations of arterial carbon dioxide

    c. is a subjective distress in breathing

    d. *a* and *b*

    e. *a*, *b*, and *c*

___ 47. Which of the following is true about overexercising?

    a. It is a recommended way to increase training volume (e.g., swimming >10,000 meters/day vs. <5,000 meters/day) and has been found to elicit a faster physiological response in aerobic capacity.

    b. It is a recommended way to increase training intensity (e.g., force on the muscle or stress on the cardiovascular system) and leads to faster improvement in conditioning response.

    c. It is not recommended, but training intensities between 40 and 85 percent of $\dot{V}O_2$max are recommended to elicit the greatest improvement in aerobic response.

    d. It is not recommended, but training at 90 percent $\dot{V}O_2$max coupled with high volume is advised for the quickest improvement in aerobic capacity.

___ 48. Of the following, what is true about overtraining?

    a. It occurs when one attempts to do more work than is physically tolerable.

    b. It usually improves physical performance at a much faster rate compared to the established training regimen.

    c. It results in anabolism proceeding at a faster rate than catabolism.

    d. *a* and *b*

    e. *a*, *b*, and *c*

___ 49. The following observations were noted in evaluating a training program for a 21-year-old female cross-country runner: increased HR at a fixed workload, unexplained poor performance, and an increased incidence of illness during the training period. What might the coach conclude about this athlete from these observations and data?

    a. She is overtraining.

    b. She requires complete rest over weeks or months.

    c. She is not training up to her capacity.

    d. *a* and *b*

    e. *a*, *b*, and *c*

___ 50. How can one prevent overuse injuries during a training regimen?

    a. Avoid large increases in training volume.

    b. Avoid large increases in training intensity.

    c. Increase training load by 10 percent (volume and intensity) per week.

    d. *a* and *b*

    e. *a*, *b*, and *c*

___ 51. To what is fatigue, as evidenced by a decrease in performance, theorized to be most likely attributed?

    a. failure of the fiber's contractile mechanism

    b. an imbalance in ATP requirement versus ATP delivery

    c. an increase in muscle acidity

    d. *a* and *b*

    e. *a*, *b*, and *c*

___ 52. Which of the following is (are) true regarding the process of glycolysis?

    a. It provides for the systematic degradation of glucose or glycogen to pyruvate.

    b. It is a predominant energy pathway during low-intensity, long-duration activity.

    c. It converts lactate to pyruvate in an anaerobic environment.

    d. *a* and *b*

    e. *a*, *b*, and *c*

___ 53. The oxidative phosphorylation of glucose involves which of the following processes?

    a. glycolysis and electron transport chain

    b. Krebs cycle and beta oxidation

    c. glycolysis, Krebs cycle, and electron transport chain

    d. *a* and *b*

___ 54. Which of the following statements is (are) true regarding the interaction of exercise intensity, duration, and energy production during activity?

    a. In efforts of two to three minutes duration, the anaerobic energy yield approximately equals the aerobic yield.

    b. In prolonged endurance activities (>10 minutes), predominant energy-producing pathways involve anaerobic metabolism.

    c. Most of the energy for performing a 400-meter dash would come from aerobic energy sources.

    d. *a*, *b*, and *c*

___ 55. Which of the following is (are) true about cardiac muscle, but *not* skeletal muscle?

    a. Cardiac muscle contains branched, striated fibers with a single nucleus.

    b. Cardiac muscle contains intercalated discs, which connect the muscle cells to function as a unit.

    c. Cardiac muscle cells can alter the force of contractions as a function of the degree of overlap between the actin and myosin filament.

d. *a* and *b*

e. *a*, *b*, and *c*

___ 56. Which of the following correctly describes the path of the heart's electrical activity?

    a. AV node, Purkinje system, atria, bundle of His, SA node, ventricles

    b. SA node, ventricles, bundle of His, AV node, Purkinje system

    c. AV node, ventricles, Purkinje system, SA node, atria, bundle of His

    d. SA node, atria, AV node, bundle of His, Purkinje system, ventricles

___ 57. In the electrocardiogram,

    a. the P wave represents atrial depolarization

    b. the T wave represents ventricular depolarization

    c. the U wave represents atrial repolarization

    d. the QRS complex represents a refractory period

___ 58. Neural regulation of the cardiovascular system during exercise demonstrates which of the following?

    a. parasympathetic withdrawal at the beginning of activity

    b. sympathetic input at higher levels of intensity

    c. changes in local metabolic conditions, causing vasodilatation in muscle

    d. *a* and *b*

    e. *a*, *b*, and *c*

___ 59. The myocardium

    a. relies on energy released from aerobic metabolism

    b. has a higher oxidative capacity compared to skeletal muscle

    c. uses primarily carbohydrates to generate ATP

    d. *a* and *b*

    e. *a*, *b*, and *c*

____ 60. Which of the following would not be considered a component of health-related physical fitness?

    a. body composition

    b. flexibility of the lower back and hamstrings

    c. aerobic fitness

    d. mental well-being

    e. abdominal muscular strength and endurance

____ 61. Flexibility

    a. is the range of motion of a given joint

    b. should be maintained in the lower back and hamstrings

    c. can be maintained through a regular stretching program

    d. *a* and *b*

    e. *a*, *b*, and *c*

____ 62. Which of the following are true concerning muscle strength and bone density?

    a. Women who maintain a strength training program can lessen their risk for fracture from osteoporosis.

    b. Women with normal bone mineral density are stronger than osteoporotic women.

    c. Postmenopausal women cannot maintain bone mineral density through resistance training.

    d. *a* and *b*

    e. *a*, *b*, and *c*

____ 63. With regard to exercise and asthma,

    a. exercise can cure asthma

    b. preexercise asthma medications will not affect exercise

    c. warm-up activities before exercise may trigger bronchospasm

    d. a cool exercise environment will benefit a person with asthma

____ 64. Which of the following factors influence the aerobic training response?

    a. initial level of fitness

b. training intensity

c. training duration

d. *a* and *b*

e. *a*, *b*, and *c*

___ 65. Isometric exercise

    a. results in a cardiovascular response due to a neurogenic mechanism

    b. results in a cardiovascular response due to a volume load on the myocardium

    c. involves an increase in systolic and diastolic blood pressures during contractions of 15 percent MVC or less

    d. *a* and *b*

    e. *a*, *b*, and *c*

___ 66. What are the physiological consequences of the Valsalva maneuver?

    a. Thoracic pressure and venous return increase.

    b. Thoracic veins collapse, reducing blood flow to the heart.

    c. It causes external straining and increases venous return.

    d. Prolonged Valsalva maneuver increases blood pressure to very dangerous levels.

___ 67. Which of the following percentage fat standards for women are accurate?

    a. obesity in young women > 35 percent

    b. athletic = 12 to 22 percent

    c. essential fat = 3 to 5 percent

    d. *a* and *b*

    e. *a*, *b*, and *c*

___ 68. Which of the following is (are) true with regard to specificity and fitness?

    a. Training effect is limited to the muscle fibers involved in the activity.

    b. Muscle fiber adapts specifically to a type of activity.

    c. Mitochondria demonstrate greater adaptation with endurance activity.

      d. *a* and *b*

      e. *a*, *b*, and *c*

___ 69. Which of the following lists of increases best demonstrates the aerobic system?

      a. key glycolytic enzymes; all-out exercise performance; mitochondrial size and number

      b. key glycolytic enzymes; capillaries of the trained muscle; mitochondrial size and number

      c. aerobic enzymes; capillaries; resting level of anaerobic substrates

      d. aerobic enzymes; oxidation of CHO; mitochondrial size and number

___ 70. The specificity principle in training is associated with which of the following?

      a. adaptations in metabolic and physiologic functions

      b. Specific exercises elicit specific training adaptations.

      c. Resistance training with high force and low repetitions will result in improved aerobic capacity and a high $\dot{V}O_2$max.

      d. *a* and *b*

      e. *a*, *b*, and *c*

___ 71. Which test(s) is (are) specific to the listed sport activity?

      a. GXT on a treadmill: running

      b. exercise test in a swim flume or a pool with a tether: swimming

      c. GXT on an arm ergometer: bicycling

      d. *a* and *b*

      e. *a*, *b*, and *c*

___ 72. In a GXT, what is the term for the power output or rate of O_2 uptake at which ventilation departs from linearity?

      a. ventilatory threshold: T_{vent}

      b. ventilatory threshold: OBLA

      c. onset of blood lactate: T_{vent}

      d. onset of blood lactate: OBLA

___ 73. The ventilatory threshold

a. results from an increase in CO_2 due to lactate buffering

b. can result in a respiratory exchange ratio to exceed 1.00

c. increases VE/VO_2

d. *a* and *b*

e. *a*, *b*, and *c*

___ 74. Maximal oxygen consumption relies on the integration of which of the following factor(s)?

a. aerobic metabolism

b. hemoglobin concentration

c. cardiac output

d. *a* and *b*

e. *a*, *b*, and *c*

___ 75. A detrained individual will demonstrate which of the following?

a. a decrease in $\dot{V}O_2$max, a decrease in a-$\bar{v}O_2$ diff max, a decrease in capillary number

b. a decrease in Q max, a decrease in HR max, capillary number unchanged

c. a decrease in a-$\bar{v}O_2$ diff max, increase in plasma volume, Q unchanged

d. a decrease in capillaries, an increase in HR max, a decrease in $\dot{V}O_2$max

___ 76. What is a commonsense guideline to follow to prevent over-training?

a. proper periodization

b. adequate recuperation during intense training cycles

c. increase fat intake during heavy training

d. *a* and *b*

e. *a*, *b*, and *c*

___ 77. Which of the following are observable signs associated with overtraining?

a. poor performance, increased fatigue, frequent infections

b. elevated resting pulse, increased injuries, disturbed mood states

  c. weight loss, depression, insomnia

  d. *a* and *b*

  e. *a*, *b*, and *c*

___ 78. Human skeletal muscle can be divided into which three fiber classifications?

  a. slow twitch, fast twitch, red and white

  b. slow twitch–oxidative (SO), fast twitch–oxidative–glycolytic (FOG), fast twitch–glycolytic (FG)

  c. type Ia, type IIb, type IIIc

  d. *a* and *b*

  e. *a*, *b*, and *c*

___ 79. Of the following, which matches the skeletal muscle fiber type to its functional characteristic?

  a. type I–slow oxidative: low force production, fatigue resistant

  b. type IIa–slow oxidative: low force production, fatigable

  c. type IIb–fast-oxidative glycolytic: high force production, fatigue resistant

  d. intermediate–fast glycolytic: high force production, fatigable

___ 80. Choose the pair(s) in which the characteristic of the fiber type matches the fiber nomenclature.

  a. oxidative metabolism: SO

  b. slow maximal shortening velocity: type I

  c. low activity of myosin-ATPase: type Iib

  d. *a* and *b*

  e. *a*, *b*, and *c*

___ 81. In the sliding filament theory of muscle contraction, actin–myosin interaction is facilitated by what two mechanisms?

  a. the release of Ca^{++} from the sarcoplasmic reticulum and the presence of ATP

  b. the attachment of ATP to troponin and myosin activation

  c. action potential initiation and the presence of ATP

  d. the release of Ca^{++} from the sarcoplasmic reticulum and the propagation of the impulse through the T tubule

___ 82. During the relaxation phase in the sliding filament theory, the following events occur. What is the correct sequence of events?

    a. The muscle returns to resting state, Ca^{++} is sequestered, actomyosin decouples, actin and myosin are recycled, ATP is resynthesized, and the nerve impulse ceases.

    b. Ca^{++} is sequestered, actin and myosin are recycled, actomyosin decouples, ATP is resynthesized, the nerve impulse ceases, and the muscle returns to resting state.

    c. ATP is resynthesized, actomyosin decouples, actin and myosin are recycled, the nerve impulse ceases, Ca^{++} is sequestered, and the muscle returns to resting state.

    d. ATP is resynthesized, actomyosin decouples, the nerve impulse ceases, actin and myosin are recycled, Ca^{++} is sequestered, and the muscle returns to resting state.

___ 83. Normal body movements involve sustained contractions and do *not* involve single muscle twitches. What is the term for normal body movements involving the addition of successive twitches, and, if the frequency of stimuli is increased further, what is this called?

    a. a submaximal response and a maximal response

    b. summation and tonus

    c. summation and tetanus

    d. tonus and tetanus

___ 84. What is true about the overload principle?

    a. It requires a progressive increase in the intensity of a workout over the course of training as fitness capacity improves.

    b. It describes a condition in which a tissue or organ is caused to work against a load that it is not accustomed to.

    c. It describes the need to increase the load in exercise to cause further adaptation of a system.

    d. *a* and *b*

    e. *a*, *b*, and *c*

____ 85. Muscle adaptations as a result of training are due to what?

    a. the principle of specificity

    b. PRE

    c. the principle of overload

    d. *a* and *b*

    e. *a*, *b*, and *c*

____ 86. Appropriate resistance training for adults includes which of the following guidelines?

    a. Use proper technique.

    b. Gradually increase resistance (approximately 5 percent).

    c. Maintain a normal breathing pattern.

    d. *a* and *b*

    e. *a*, *b*, and *c*

____ 87. What is the number of repetitions and sets recommended to predominantly increase muscle strength?

    a. performing between 3RM and 12RM

    b. PRE training once weekly with 1RM; 1 set

    c. PRE; multiple exercise; two to three days per week

    d. *a* and *b*

    e. *a*, *b*, and *c*

____ 88. Which of the following are true with regard to strength training in the healthy adult?

    a. Perform at least 8 to 10 separate exercises; minimum of one set; two to three d/wk.

    b. Perform 10 to 15 repetitions for development of muscular endurance.

    c. The healthy adult should never train with "free weights" because technique is difficult and safety is an issue.

    d. *a* and *b*

    e. *a*, *b*, and *c*

____ 89. Choose the pair(s) in which the abnormal condition is matched with the appropriate normal symptom.

    a. dyspnea: 12 breaths per minute at rest

b. orthostatic hypotension: 120/80 mmHg

c. PVC: bradycardia

d. *a* and *b*

e. *a*, *b*, and *c*

___ 90. Which statement is true about exercise and blood pressure?

    a. Exercise must be terminated when SBP reaches 190 mmHg.

    b. Exertional hypotension has been correlated with myocardial ischemia and left ventricular dysfunction.

    c. There is a linear increase in DBP with increasing levels of exercise.

    d. Automated blood pressure devices provide a more accurate assessment of SBP and DBP during an exercise test.

___ 91. Static exercise or activities that involve high resistance cause what changes in SBP and DBP, respectively?

    a. progressive increase; no change or slight decrease

    b. at <20 percent MVC increase; no change

    c. at >20 percent MVC increase; increase

    d. at >50 percent MVC; neither SBP nor DBP can be determined at this intensity

___ 92. Body inversion techniques used to facilitate a strength-training response or relieve low back pain cause what changes in SBP and DBP, respectively?

    a. increase; decrease

    b. increase; increase

    c. decrease; no change

    d. decrease; decrease

___ 93. Which of the following is (are) indicative of a hypertensive BP response?

    a. stage 1: SBP > 160 mmHg; DBP > 90 mmHg

    b. stage 2: SBP < 120 mmHg; DBP < 100 mmHg

    c. stage 3: SBP > 180 mmHg; DBP > 110 mmHg

    d. stage 4: SBP > 200 mmHg; DBP < 100 mmHg

___ 94. One may be at risk for type 2 diabetes if

    a. one is a member of a high risk ethnic group

    b. one delivered a baby weighing more than nine pounds

    c. one has a first degree relative with diabetes (genetic influence)

    d. *a* and *b*

    e. *a, b,* and *c*

___ 95. Which of the following changes in skeletal muscle results from anaerobic training?

    a. a decrease in the capacity of the phosphagen system

    b. a decrease in the muscular stores of ATP and PC

    c. a slower ATP turnover rate

    d. an increase in glycolytic enzyme activities

___ 96. What changes at rest are induced by training?

    a. increased size of the left atrial cavity in endurance athletes

    b. decrease in left ventricular wall thickness in non-endurance athletes

    c. decrease in the intrinsic atrial HR in endurance athletes

    d. decrease in parasympathetic tone

___ 97. What changes occurring during maximal work are influenced by endurance training?

    a. increase in $\dot{V}O_2$max; increase in Q max

    b. increase in HR max; increase in SV max

    c. increase in sympathetic drive; increase in intrinsic pacemaker rate

    d. decrease in lactate production; decrease in blood flow per kilogram of active muscle

___ 98. What causes cardiac output (Q) to increase during acute exercise?

    a. a rise in HR; an increase in SV

    b. a rise in BP; an increase in peripheral resistance

    c. a rise in HR; an increase in venous return

    d. an increase in SV; a decrease in parasympathetic tone

___ 99. What is the reason for the increase in ventilation ($\dot{V}_E$) during acute exercise?

    a. increase in $\dot{V}O_2$ and blood pressure

    b. increase in tidal volume and frequency of breathing

    c. increase in peripheral resistance and $\dot{V}O_2$

    d. increase in frequency of breathing and vital capacity

___100. Exercise training can benefit those with type 1 diabetes in which of the following ways?

    a. lowering body fat

    b. increasing peripheral sensitivity to insulin

    c. increasing glucose intolerance

    d. *a* and *b*

    e. *a*, *b*, and *c*

___101. Proteins that can be found in a muscle fiber include

    a. actin and myosin

    b. troponin and tropomyosin

    c. M and C proteins

    d. *a* and *b*

    e. *a*, *b*, and *c*

___102. The structural entity that makes up the functional unit of a muscle fiber is the

    a. fasiculi

    b. sarcomere

    c. sarcoplasmic reticulum

    d. *a* and *b*

    e. *a*, *b*, and *c*

___103. A sudden increase in blood lactate levels equal to 4.0 mM

    a. is termed anaerobic threshold

    b. is termed lactate threshold

    c. is termed OBLA

    d. *a* and *b*

    e. *a*, *b*, and *c*

____104. Arrhythmia

    a. is also called dysrhythmia

    b. can cause tachycardia or bradycardia

    c. appears in 1 out of every 100 births

    d. *a* and *b*

    e. *a*, *b*, and *c*

____105. Essential components in an exercise prescription should include

    a. appropriate exercise mode for the individual

    b. a calculation of the appropriate intensity, frequency, and duration

    c. $\dot{V}O_2max$

    d. *a* and *b*

    e. *a*, *b*, and *c*

____106. Which of the following are possible maximal stroke volume measurements during graded exercise?

    a. 184 ml/beat in a world-class runner

    b. 35 L/min in a world-class runner

    c. 16.0 ml/dl of blood in a world-class runner

    d. *a* and *b*

    e. *a*, *b*, and *c*

____107. Evaluate the following statement: Stroke volume increases linearly with graded exercise until it reaches approximately 50 percent of aerobic capacity.

    a. true for unconditioned individuals

    b. true for athletes

    c. true among healthy adults

    d. *a* and *b*

    e. *a*, *b*, and *c*

____108. The fatigue associated with short-duration, high-intensity exercise is due to

    a. decreasing pH, which reduces maximal tension in skeletal and cardiac muscle

    b. an increase in the threshold of free calcium, which is required for contraction

    c. glycogen depletion

    d. *a* and *b*

    e. *a*, *b*, and *c*

___109. Low-frequency fatigue is characterized by

    a. a disruption of the E–C coupling process

    b. prolonged recovery

    c. inadequate neural drive by the motor cortex

    d. *a* and *b*

    e. *a*, *b*, and *c*

___110. Which of the following statement(s) is (are) true for premature atrial contractions (PACs)?

    a. They occur when a site in the atrium other than the sinus node depolarizes prematurely.

    b. They generate a narrow QRS complex.

    c. They are not uncommon during exercise testing when catecholamine levels are increased.

    d. *a* and *b*

    e. *a*, *b*, and *c*

REFERENCES FOR FURTHER STUDY

1. ACSM. (2001). *ACSM's resource manual for guidelines for exercise testing and prescription* (4th ed.). Philadelphia: Lippincott Williams & Wilkins.

2. ACSM. (2000). *ACSM's guidelines for exercise testing and prescription* (6th ed.). Philadelphia: Lippincott Williams & Wilkins.

3. McArdle, W.D., Katch, F.I., & Katch, V.I. (2001). *Exercise physiology: Energy, nutrition, and human performance* (5th ed.). Baltimore: Williams & Wilkins.

ANSWERS

Question number	Answer	KSA number	Reference	Page number
1	b	1.2.1	3	133
2	d	1.2.1	3	135, 138
3	a	1.2.2	3	164
4	c	1.2.2	3	164
5	d	1.2.3	1	143
			3	345
6	b	1.2.3	3	160
7	d	1.2.3	3	265
8	a	1.2.3	3	308
9	b	1.2.3	3	308
10	e	1.2.3	1	240
11	e	1.2.3	3	329, 929
12	d	1.2.3	3	331
13	e	1.2.3	3	321
14	a	1.2.3	3	320
15	a	1.2.4	3	14, 16
16	d	1.2.5	2	145
17	d	1.2.5	2	160
18	a	1.2.5	2	158
19	e	1.2.5	1	398
			2	64
20	b	1.2.9	3	334
21	a	2.2.13	1	427

Question number	Answer	KSA number	Reference	Page number
22	d	1.2.6	3	242, 319
23	d	1.2.6	3	233
24	c	1.2.6	1	147
25	d	1.2.6	1	147
26	e	1.2.6	3	167
27	e	1.2.7	3	464, 472-473
28	a	1.2.7	1	161
29	e	1.2.7	3	471
30	d	1.2.8	3	532
31	e	1.2.8	3	530
32	d	1.2.8	3	530
33	d	1.2.8	3	537
34	d	1.2.8	3	531
35	a	1.2.8	3	530
36	b	1.2.8	3	531, 536
37	b	1.2.9	1	364
38	e	1.2.10	3	574
39	e	1.2.10	3	574
40	e	1.2.10	3	170, 316
41	b	1.2.10	3	574
42	e	1.2.10	1	451
43	e	2.2.17	1	217
44	d	2.2.17	3	607, 614
45	e	2.2.17	3	265

Question number	Answer	KSA number	Reference	Page number
46	e	2.2.17	3	265
47	c	2.2.21	2	145
48	a	2.2.21	3	489-491
49	d	2.2.21	3	491
50	e	2.2.21	3	489-491
51	e	1.2.11	3	400-402
52	a	1.2.1	3	141-143
53	c	1.2.1	3	137
54	a	1.2.2	1	133-135
55	d	2.2.10	3	308
56	d	2.2.10	3	326
57	a	2.2.10	3	329
58	e	2.2.10	3	330
59	d	2.2.10	3	322
60	d	2.2.18	1	489
61	e	2.2.18	2	156
62	d	2.2.18	3	538
63	b	2.2.22	3	957
64	e	2.2.18	3	478
65	a	2.2.12	1	147
66	b	2.2.12	3	265
67	d	2.2.18	1	398
68	e	2.2.19	1	484
69	d	2.2.1	3	466

Question number	Answer	KSA number	Reference	Page number
70	d	2.2.19	3	460-463
71	d	2.2.19	1	489
72	a	2.2.15	3	291
73	e	2.2.15	3	291, 293
74	e	2.2.0	3	161
75	d	2.2.20	3	464
			1	191
76	d	2.2.21	3	491
77	e	2.2.21	3	491
78	b	2.2.4	3	375
79	a	2.2.4	3	375
80	d	2.2.4	3	375
81	a	2.2.5	3	372
82	c	2.2.5	3	374
83	c	2.2.6	1	87
84	e	2.2.7	1	449
85	e	2.2.7	1	461
86	e	2.2.9	1	463
87	d	2.2.9	3	511
88	d	2.2.9	2	160
89	d	2.2.17	1	656
90	b	2.2.14	1	143
91	c	2.2.14	1	147
92	b	2.2.14	3	320

Question number	Answer	KSA number	Reference	Page number
93	c	2.2.22	1	286
94	e	2.2.22	3	433
95	d	2.2.1	3	464
96	c	2.2.1	3	464, 466
97	a	2.2.1	3	466
98	a	2.2.11	1	143
99	b	2.2.11	1	144
100	d	2.2.22	1	277
101	e	2.2.3	3	362
102	b	2.2.3	3	362
103	c	1.2.3	3	291
104	d	1.2.3	3	928
105	d	1.2.0	2	139
106	a	2.2.2	1	144
107	e	2.2.2	1	142
108	d	2.2.8	1	186
109	d	2.2.8	1	187
110	e	2.2.13	1	427

6

Human Development and Aging

In this category, Human Development and Aging, you will be required to answer approximately eight questions. Emphasis is placed on your ability to distinguish differences between young children and older adults relative to unique adaptations to exercise, differences in exercise prescription, and the developmental effects of aging on physiological fitness.

PRACTICE QUESTIONS

Instructions: Each question is followed by either four or five possible answers. Select the *best* answer to the question.

_____ 1. Children are less able than adults to thermoregulate during heat exposure because children exhibit which of the following characteristics?

   a. lower threshold for the onset of sweating, lower skin blood flow, higher sweat output from heat-activated sweat glands, and smaller surface area to body mass ratio

   b. lower threshold for the onset of sweating, higher skin blood flow, lower sweat output from heat-activated sweat glands, and smaller surface area to body mass ratio

   c. higher threshold for the onset of sweating, lower skin blood flow, lower sweat output from heat-activated sweat glands, and larger surface area to body mass ratio

d. higher threshold for the onset of sweating, higher skin blood flow, higher sweat output from heat-activated sweat glands, and larger surface area to body mass ratio

___ 2. At what rate do women over the age of 35 tend to lose bone mass?

    a. .05 percent per year

    b. 1.0 percent per year

    c. 1.5 percent per year

    d. 2.0 percent per year

___ 3. Within an elderly population, what change occurs in resting HR?

    a. decrease

    b. increase

    c. little to no change

    d. increase in men but decrease in women

    e. increase in women but decrease in men

___ 4. As people age, what change occurs in maximal HR?

    a. decrease

    b. increase

    c. little to no change

    d. increase in men but decrease in women

    e. increase in women but decrease in men

___ 5. Peak flexibility, as measured by the sit-and-reach test, is generally obtained at what age?

    a. prior to 10 years of age

    b. between 12 and 15 years of age

    c. during the late teens and early 20s

    d. between 30 and 35 years of age

___ 6. By 65 years of age, what is the approximate decline in muscular function?

    a. 5 percent

    b. 10 percent

   c. 15 percent

   d. 25 percent

___ 7. $\dot{V}O_2$max in adulthood declines at about what rate per year?

   a. 0.5 percent

   b. 1.0 percent

   c. 1.5 percent

   d. 2.0 percent

___ 8. Excessive endurance exercise in a prepubescent child could place the child at increased risk for what problem?

   a. a decrease in height

   b. an epiphyseal growth plate injury

   c. rotator cuff injury

   d. none of the above

___ 9. What is the minimum stage or age a child should reach before being permitted to perform maximum lifts (1RM)?

   a. 10 years of age

   b. 18 years of age

   c. Tanner stage 3 level of maturity

   d. Tanner stage 5 level of maturity

___ 10. What is true about elderly individuals who regularly participate in a resistance-training program?

   a. Significant increases occur in muscle cross-sectional area within the first six weeks of training.

   b. They tend to be more self-sufficient.

   c. They tend to perform daily living skills with greater ease.

   d. They show no physiological advantage over peers who maintain a sedentary lifestyle.

   e. *b* and *c*

___ 11. The exercise leader should be aware of leadership techniques that meet the needs of special populations. Which of the following pertain(s) especially to young children from special populations engaged in an exercise program?

   a. frequent change of activity

b. frequent rest periods

c. frequent use of demonstrations

d. *a* and *b*

e. *a*, *b*, and *c*

____ 12. At maximal intensities, how much lower is the cardiac output of older adults than that of younger individuals?

a. 1 to 5 percent

b. 10 to 20 percent

c. 20 to 30 percent

d. 30 to 40 percent

____ 13. What change occurs in residual volume by 70 years of age?

a. It decreases by 5 to 10 percent.

b. It decreases by 30 to 50 percent.

c. It increases by 5 to 10 percent.

d. It increases by 30 to 50 percent.

____ 14. Which of the following decrease(s) with age?

a. size of muscle fibers

b. number of muscle fibers

c. maximal HR

d. *a* and *c*

e. *a*, *b*, and *c*

____ 15. ACSM guidelines recommend, for young, healthy individuals, an exercise intensity that is between 50 and 85 percent of HRR. What is the recommended percentage for older adults?

a. 50 to 60 percent of HRR

b. 50 to 60 percent of HR max

c. 50 to 70 percent of HRR

d. talk test is used to monitor exercise intensity

____ 16. In comparison to the ACSM guideline recommending that young children perform resistance-training exercise no more than two days per week, what is recommended for elderly individuals?

a. daily

b. one day per week

c. two days per week

d. three days per week

e. five days per week

___ 17. What increase, if any, is demonstrated by older adults who participate regularly in a strength-training program?

a. increased strength in the absence of muscle hypertrophy

b. increased strength with moderate muscle hypertrophy

c. increased strength with significant muscle hypertrophy

d. little to no increase in muscle strength

___ 18. What increase, if any, is generally demonstrated in prepubescent children who regularly participate in a weight-training program?

a. increased strength in the absence of muscle hypertrophy

b. increased strength with moderate muscle hypertrophy

c. increased strength with significant muscle hypertrophy

d. little to no increase in muscular strength

___ 19. Of the following, what is the most appropriate exercise modification for an elderly individual with degenerative joint disease?

a. bench stepping

b. stair climbing

c. stationary cycling

d. running

___ 20. What is the most appropriate exercise modification for an elderly individual with hypertension?

a. emphasis on high-resistance, low-repetition, isotonic training

b. emphasis on high-resistance, high-repetition, isotonic training

c. emphasis on low-resistance, low-repetition, isotonic training

d. emphasis on isometric training

____ 21. What adjustment should be made by the elderly individual who is engaged in resistance training during periods of arthritic pain?

     a. Reduce training from two days per week to one day per week.

     b. Reduce training from three days per week to two days per week.

     c. Reduce exercise intensity and increase the number of repetitions.

     d. Reduce both exercise intensity and number of repetitions.

     e. Avoid resistance training during periods of pain.

____ 22. After a lay-off from resistance training exercise, it is recommended that the elderly individual first use an exercise intensity of this percent of the 1RM:

     a. 90

     b. 80

     c. 70

     d. 60

     e. 50

____ 23. Of the following cardiovascular-related statements, which is most appropriate for an inactive elderly individual?

     a. Run 30 minutes on most days of the week.

     b. Accumulate 30 minutes of activity on most days with the activity broken into three 10-minute sessions.

     c. Perform 30 minutes of vigorous activity four days per week.

     d. Become involved on an adult basketball league competing for 30 minutes on most days of the week.

REFERENCES FOR FURTHER STUDY

1. ACSM. (1993). *ACSM's resource manual for guidelines for exercise testing and prescription* (2nd ed.). Malvern, PA: Lea & Febiger.

2. ACSM. (2001). *ACSM's resource manual for guidelines for exercise testing and prescription* (4th ed.). Philadelphia: Lippincott Williams & Wilkins.

3. ACSM. (2000). *ACSM's guidelines for exercise testing and prescription* (6th ed.). Philadelphia: Lippincott Williams & Wilkins.

4. Payne, V.G., & Isaacs, L.D. (2002). *Human motor development: A lifespan approach* (5th ed.). Boston: McGraw-Hill.

ANSWERS

Question number	Answer	KSA number	Reference	Page number
1	c	2.3.0.2	2	522
2	b	2.3.0.2	2	515
3	c	2.3.0.2	3	223
4	a	2.3.0.2	3	223
5	c	2.3.0.2	4	192
6	d	2.3.0.2	2	515
7	b	2.3.0.2	4	179
8	b	1.3.0	2	523
9	d	1.3.0	4	188
10	e	1.3.1	3	227
11	e	1.3.2	1	325
12	c	2.3.0.3	1	418
13	d	2.3.0.3	1	419
14	e	2.3.0.3	4	191
15	d	2.3.0.4	2	531
16	c	2.3.0.4	3	228
17	b	2.3.0.5	4	189-191
18	a	2.3.0.5	4	190
19	c	2.3.0.6	3	224

Question number	Answer	KSA number	Reference	Page number
20	c	2.3.0.6	3	228
21	e	2.3.0.6	3	229
22	e	2.3.0.1	3	228
23	b	2.3.0.1	3	227

Pathophysiology and Risk Factors

We suggest that you begin your study of this ACSM KSA category, Pathophysiology and Risk Factors, by first memorizing the CAD risk factors listed on page 24 of *ACSM's Guidelines for Exercise Testing and Prescription* (ACSM, 2000). You will be required to answer approximately 10 questions from this category.

PRACTICE QUESTIONS

Instructions: Each question is followed by either four or five possible answers. Select the *best* answer to the question.

_____ 1. What change in cholesterol is associated with an increase in physical activity?

    a. an increase in LDL-C

    b. an increase in HDL-C

    c. an increase in both HDL-C and LDL-C

    d. a decrease in both HDL-C and LDL-C

_____ 2. A reduction in dietary sodium intake, weight reduction, and an increase in physical activity will generally allow a patient to modify which of the following CAD risk factors?

    a. hypercholesterolemia

    b. hypertension

    c. diabetes mellitus

    d. VLDL-C

___ 3. Of the following cholesterol measures, which is the best determinant of CAD risk?

    a. TC : HDL-C ratio

    b. HDL-C : LDL-C ratio

    c. TC

    d. LDL-C : VLDL-C ratio

___ 4. In the mild (stage 1) hypertensive, what would be the expected range for adult resting SBP and DBP, respectively?

    a. 130 to 139 mmHg; 85 to 90 mmHg

    b. 140 to 159 mmHg; 90 to 99 mmHg

    c. 160 to 179 mmHg; 100 to 109 mmHg

    d. 180 to 209 mmHg; 110 to 119 mmHg

___ 5. In the moderate (stage 2) hypertensive, what would be the expected range of adult resting SBP and DBP, respectively?

    a. 130 to 139 mmHg; 85 to 90 mmHg

    b. 140 to 159 mmHg; 90 to 99 mmHg

    c. 160 to 179 mmHg; 100 to 109 mmHg

    d. 180 to 209 mmHg; 110 to 119 mmHg

___ 6. What procedure should be followed when SBP and DBP fall into different classification categories?

    a. Classify according to the higher category.

    b. Classify according to the lower category.

    c. Do not classify at this time, but continue to retest weekly until both SBP and DBP measures fall within the same category.

    d. Do not classify at this time, but continue to retest every six weeks until both SBP and DBP measures fall within the same category.

___ 7. Which of the following, if any, is (are) true regarding hypertension?

    a. Hypertension is more prevalent among women and whites than among men and blacks.

    b. Primary hypertension is caused by identifiable endocrine or structural disorders.

   c. One is hypertensive if exercise BP > 129/84 mmHg.

   d. All of these are true statements.

   e. None of these are true statements.

___ 8. What lipoprotein is the primary carrier of serum cholesterol?

   a. HDL-C

   b. LDL-C

   c. VLDL-C

   d. triglyceride

___ 9. What lipoprotein is primarily responsible for transporting cholesterol out of the system?

   a. VLDL-C

   b. LDL-C

   c. HDL-C

   d. triglyceride

___ 10. What causes anemia?

   a. decrease in red blood cell production

   b. increase in red blood cell production

   c. increase in red blood cell destruction

   d. blood loss

   e. *a, c,* and *d*

___ 11. Which of the following is the most desirable TC : HDL-C ratio?

   a. TC 199 : HDL-C 38

   b. TC 190 : HDL-C 50

   c. TC 210 : HDL-C 62

   d. TC 175 : HDL-C 36

___ 12. What can result from a mismatch between active muscle O_2 supply and demand?

   a. ischemic pain

   b. claudication

   c. tightness or cramping

   d. *a* and *b*

   e. *a, b,* and *c*

____ 13. Given the following health information, which abnormal findings for a 34-year-old male would require consultation with a physician or allied health professional prior to granting exercise clearance? Resting BP = 130/96; resting HR = 72 beats per minute; TC = 210; LDL-C = 155 mg/dl; HDL-C = 42 mg/dl

    a. BP, TC, and HDL-C are too high.

    b. BP, TC, and LDL-C are too high while HDL-C is too low.

    c. BP, TC, LDL-C are too low while HDL-C is too high.

    d. BP, TC, and LDL-C are too high.

____ 14. What should the exercise professional recommend to a client who indicates a desire to increase exercise intensity because she believes her sudden breathlessness during mild exertion is a matter of not pushing herself hard enough?

    a. Increase the exercise intensity by five percent.

    b. Increase the exercise duration from 30 to 45 minutes but maintain the current level of exercise intensity.

    c. Decrease the exercise duration from 30 to 15 minutes and increase exercise intensity by 20 percent.

    d. Require the client to consult with his physician before proceeding with any exercise program.

____ 15. Which symptom(s) is (are) associated with asthma?

    a. wheezing

    b. nonproductive cough

    c. productive cough in which sputum is produced

    d. *a* and *b*

    e. *a* and *c*

____ 16. Which symptom(s) is (are) associated with bronchitis?

    a. wheezing

    b. nonproductive cough

    c. productive cough in which sputum is produced

    d. *a* and *b*

    e. *a* and *c*

___ 17. A positive test for exercise-induced asthma is noted when there is what percent of reduction in forced expiratory volume in one second following an exercise challenge?

    a. 5

    b. 10

    c. 15

    d. 20

    e. 25

___ 18. Is there a need for a male with the following preexercise test evaluation to consult with a medical professional before participating in a physical activity program? 20 years of age; weight = 62 kilograms; hemoglobin = 14 g/dl; fasting glucose = 205 mg/dl; HDL-C = 42 mg/dl; LDL-C = 120 mg/dl; SBP = 138 mmHg; DBP = 83 mmHg

    a. No, all values are within appropriate ranges.

    b. Yes, HDL-C is too low.

    c. Yes, fasting glucose is too high.

    d. Yes, there are signs of anemia.

    e. *c* and *d*

___ 19. What should the exercise professional do with regard to a client who wishes to begin a jogging program geared to strengthening the muscles in her painful lower back?

    a. Have the client perform the Cooper 1.5-mile run before recommending a specific exercise program.

    b. Instruct the client to run only on a soft indoor track.

    c. Show the client how to do back hyperextension exercises in order to strengthen the lower back before starting a jogging program.

    d. Require the client to consult her personal physician before starting an exercise program.

    e. Instruct the client to engage in bed rest for three weeks before starting a jogging program.

___ 20. Aggressive CAD risk factor management following an MI may

    a. reduce the vulnerability to plaque rupture

    b. stabilize plaque in the absence of atherosclerotic regression

    c. normalize endothelial function

    d. *a* and *b*

    e. *a*, *b*, and *c*

___ 21. Vascular endothelial dysfunction can likely lead to which of the following?

    a. impaired vasodilation

    b. decreased permeability to lipoproteins

    c. decreased thrombogenesis

    d. *b* and *c*

    e. *a*, *b*, and *c*

___ 22. Weight gain has been shown to be an important predictor of increased cholesterol. Which of the following represents a true target exercise guideline for improving lipids?

    a. Do aerobic exercise two days per week.

    b. Minimum kilocalories per week expended by exercise should be between 1,000 and 1,200.

    c. With aerobic exercise, target lipids levels can be reached within three months.

    d. Aerobic exercise intensity should be between 30 percent and 40 percent of maximal exercise capacity.

___ 23. According to the American Heart Association's dietary therapy recommendations for treating abnormal lipids, the Step I diet should contain less than this percent of calories from fat:

    a. 10

    b. 15

    c. 20

    d. 25

    e. 30

___ 24. What is the term for an inflammatory disorder affecting the sac lying between muscle and bone?

    a. bursitis

    b. tendinitis

    c. plantar fasciitis

    d. myositis

____ 25. What is the term for an inflammatory disorder of muscles and/or tendons that attach at the elbow joint?

    a. capsulitis

    b. epicondylitis

    c. bursitis

    d. synovitis

____ 26. What is the term for an inflammatory disorder of the fibrous tissue that attaches muscle to bone?

    a. bursitis

    b. capsulitis

    c. synovitis

    d. tendinitis

____ 27. Which of the following is the definition of osteoporosis?

    a. an inflammatory disease of the joints that affects only older adults

    b. an inflammatory disease of the joints that can affect young and old alike

    c. a loss of bone mass resulting in bone thinning and bone weakening

    d. a loss of serotonin

____ 28. What is the term for an inflammatory joint condition with an underlying autoimmune component?

    a. osteoarthritis

    b. osteoporosis

    c. chondromalacia

    d. rheumatoid arthritis

    e. *a* and *d*

____ 29. Which of the following refers to the softening of cartilage?

    a. chondromalacia

    b. osteoporosis

c. tendinitis

d. cardiomyopathy

___ 30. Which of the following factors is (are) believed to contribute to coronary artery injury?

a. hypercholesterolemia

b. hypertension

c. viral infections

d. *a* and *b*

e. *a*, *b*, and *c*

___ 31. How does exercise influence the atherosclerotic process?

a. It decreases HDL-C, increases triglycerides, and decreases BP.

b. It increases HDL-C, increases triglycerides, and decreases BP.

c. It increases HDL-C, decreases triglycerides, and increases BP.

d. It increases HDL-C, decreases triglycerides, and decreases BP.

REFERENCES FOR FURTHER STUDY

1. ACSM. (2001). *ACSM's resource manual for guidelines for exercise testing and prescription* (4th ed.). Philadelphia: Lippincott Williams & Wilkins.
2. ACSM. (2000). *ACSM's guidelines for exercise testing and prescription* (6th ed.). Philadelphia: Lippincott Williams & Wilkins.
3. Anderson, K.N. (Ed.) (1994). *Mosby's medical, nursing, and allied health dictionary* (4th ed.). St. Louis: Mosby.
4. Baechle, T.R., & Earle, R.W. (Eds.) (2000). *Essentials of strength training and conditioning* (2nd ed.). Champaign, IL: Human Kinetics.
5. Howley, E.T., & Franks, B.D. (2003). *Health fitness instructor's handbook* (4th ed.). Champaign, IL: Human Kinetics.

ANSWERS

Question number	Answer	KSA number	Reference	Page number
1	b	1.4.0.1	1	311
2	b	1.4.0.1	2	207
3	a	1.4.0.1	5	36
		1.4.0.1	4	219
4	b	1.4.0.2	2	41
5	c	1.4.0.2	2	41
6	a	1.4.0.2	2	41
7	e	1.4.0.2	2	206
8	b	1.4.0.2	1	308
9	c	1.4.0.2	1	308
10	e	1.4.0.2	3	84
11	c	1.4.0.3	5	36
12	e	2.4.4	2	208-209
13	d	2.4.4	2	41, 44-47
14	d	2.4.5	2	25
15	d	2.4.5	1	332
16	e	2.4.5	1	328
17	c	2.4.5	2	131
18	c	2.4.6	2	48
19	d	2.4.7	1	120-128
20	e	2.4.1	1	268
21	a	2.4.2	1	228
22	b	2.4.2	1	314

Question number	Answer	KSA number	Reference	Page number
23	e	2.4.3	1	313
24	a	2.4.7	5	410
25	b	2.4.7	5	410
26	d	2.4.7	5	410
27	c	2.4.7	1	299
28	a	2.4.7	3	1368
29	a	2.4.7	3	324
30	e	2.4.0	1	228
31	d	2.4.3	1	313

8

Human Behavior and Psychology

The emphasis of this ACSM KSA category, Human Behavior and Psychology, is effective communication primarily for the purpose of changing health behaviors. It is essential that the Health/Fitness Instructor know how to deal effectively with various personalities when implementing programs designed to improve exercise adherence as well as other targeted health behaviors, such as those related to smoking, diet, and stress management. You are likely to receive five questions from this category. We suggest that you begin your study of this KSA category by consulting chapter 12 in *ACSM's Guidelines for Exercise Testing and Prescription, Sixth Edition* (ACSM, 2000).

PRACTICE QUESTIONS

Instructions: Each question is followed by either four or five possible answers. Select the *best* answer to the question.

_____ 1. Which of the following elements should be a part of each health counseling session?

    a. acceptance

    b. expressing empathy

    c. assessing health-related behavior

    d. *a* and *b*

    e. *a*, *b*, and *c*

___ 2. Nonverbal communication is a skill each health counselor should develop. This would include which of the following elements?

    a. kinesics: body movements that convey information

    b. paralinguistics: characteristics of personal space

    c. proxemics: characteristics of speech

    d. *a* and *b*

    e. *a*, *b*, and *c*

___ 3. Change in health and exercise behavior is successful when which of the following components are included in a program?

    a. set short- and long-term, realistic, and measurable goals

    b. have client sign a contract with a description of the goal and how the goal is to be achieved

    c. provide frequent feedback on client's success

    d. *a* and *b*

    e. *a*, *b*, and *c*

___ 4. What term is used to identify any action implemented during or after the occurrence of a behavior that increases the probability that the behavior will occur again?

    a. goal-setting

    b. reinforcement

    c. shaping

    d. stimulus–control

___ 5. What is the term for a health behavior-change strategy that recognizes the need to change health behavior gradually?

    a. cognitive behavior

    b. contracting

    c. shaping

    d. self-management

___ 6. People are motivated to begin an exercise program for a variety of reasons. Which of the following may aid in this motivation process?

    a. role models

    b. information on "how to make a change" written at a seventh grade level or below

    c. previous experience that found a health behavior change beneficial

    d. *a* and *b*

    e. *a*, *b*, and *c*

___ 7. Which of the reinforcement applications would be considered intrinsic in nature?

    a. praise from an exercise leader

    b. receiving a certificate or patch after reaching a goal

    c. individual accomplishment and increasing self-confidence

    d. *a* and *b*

    e. *a*, *b*, and *c*

___ 8. Which of these recommendations would be motivating for the exercise participant?

    a. physician support in the exercise program

    b. exercising with others

    c. periodic testing

    d. *a* and *b*

    e. *a*, *b*, and *c*

___ 9. Which of the following stages of *motivational readiness* is matched with the correct definition?

    a. precontemplation: patients have been in action for six months or more

    b. action: patients express lack of interest in making change

    c. contemplation: patients are thinking about making a change

    d. preparation: patients have not maintained the appropriate behavior changes

___ 10. Which exercise performance awards are extrinsic in nature?

    a. jogging a total of 100 miles in three months and receiving a free t-shirt

    b. a good feeling of accomplishment for having jogged 100 miles in three months

    c. a good feeling of accomplishment for having lost four pounds in one month

    d. a good feeling of accomplishment for increasing HDL-C by 5 mg/dl

___ 11. Which of the following counseling approaches may assist the less-motivated client to exercise?

    a. social cognitive theory

    b. behavior modification

    c. generalization training theory

    d. *a* and *b*

    e. *a*, *b*, and *c*

___ 12. Which of the following counseling approaches would assist a less-motivated client to exercise?

    a. Discuss a plan of action.

    b. Develop a plan of action.

    c. Agree on a plan of action.

    d. *a* and *b*

    e. *a*, *b*, and *c*

___ 13. Adherence to an exercise program is enhanced by which of the following factors?

    a. convenience

    b. behavioral shaping

    c. enjoyability

    d. *a* and *b*

    e. *a*, *b*, and *c*

___ 14. Which of the following health behavioral change strategies is (are) useful for helping a client maintain exercise adherence?

    a. using a written contract

    b. before the client engages in an exercise program, requiring him/her to develop an exercise relapse prevention program

    c. making the participant feel guilty if he/she contemplates stopping the exercise program

d. *a* and *b*

e. *a*, *b*, and *c*

___ 15. Which of the following approaches to the health behavior change model are sequenced correctly?

    a. adoption, antecedents, maintenance

    b. antecedents, information, instruction

    c. antecedents, adoption, maintenance

    d. information, instruction, information

___ 16. Depression

    a. affects 5 to 10 percent of all adults during their lifetimes

    b. is common after myocardial infarction

    c. requires hospitalization

    d. *a* and *b*

    e. *a*, *b*, and *c*

___ 17. What are the symptoms of depression?

    a. feeling blue

    b. sometimes having suicidal feelings

    c. fatigue or trouble sleeping

    d. *a* and *b*

    e. *a*, *b*, and *c*

___ 18. Which of the following are considered anxiety disorders?

    a. generalized anxiety disorder

    b. panic disorder

    c. social phobia

    d. *a* and *b*

    e. *a*, *b*, and *c*

___ 19. Which of the following anxiety disorders is (are) correctly matched with the appropriate description?

    a. generalized anxiety disorder: fear of social situations

    b. panic disorder: periods of apprehension or fear

    c. social phobia: excessive worry, trembling, and muscle tension

    d. *a* and *b*

    e. *a*, *b*, and *c*

___ 20. Which of the following physiological symptoms might indicate test anxiety in a client?

    a. high resting heart rate

    b. high resting blood pressure

    c. muscle pain

    d. *a* and *b*

    e. *a*, *b*, and *c*

___ 21. Which of the following is a (are) good way(s) to relieve test anxiety in a client?

    a. Explain the test thoroughly to the client.

    b. Demonstrate the safe use of the treadmill or other testing device.

    c. Answer all the client's questions.

    d. *a* and *b*

    e. *a*, *b*, and *c*

REFERENCES FOR FURTHER STUDY

1. ACSM. (2001). *ACSM's resource manual for guidelines for exercise testing and prescription* (4th ed.). Philadelphia: Lippincott Williams & Wilkins.

2. ACSM. (2000). *ACSM's guidelines for exercise testing and prescription* (6th ed.). Philadelphia: Lippincott Williams & Wilkins.

ANSWERS

Question number	Answer	KSA number	Reference	Page number
1	e	1.5.1	1	537
2	a	1.5.1	1	538
3	e	1.5.0	2	241
4	b	1.5.0	1	559

Question number	Answer	KSA number	Reference	Page number
5	c	1.5.0	2	243
6	e	1.5.2	1	557
7	c	1.5.2	2	243
			1	559, 580
8	e	1.5.2	2	245
9	c	1.5.3	2	242
10	a	1.5.2	1	580
11	d	1.5.4	2	241
12	e	1.5.4	1	539
13	e	2.5.0	1	579
14	d	2.5.0	1	581
15	c	2.5.0	1	557
16	d	2.5.1	1	551
17	e	2.5.1	1	553
18	e	2.5.1	1	551
19	b	2.5.1	1	551
20	d	2.5.2	2	254
21	e	2.5.2	2	59
			1	367

CHAPTER

9

Health Appraisal and Fitness Testing

The ACSM KSA category *Health Appraisal and Fitness Testing* consists of four general and 26 specific objectives. You will likely encounter 10 questions from this category. To obtain a passing score, it is mandatory that you commit to memory most of the information we present in table 1.2 (see chapter 1). Pay particular attention to the information regarding informed consent, absolute and relative indications for terminating an exercise test, recommendations for medical exam and exercise testing before participation, and recommendations for physician supervision of an exercise test, as well as information related to individual test procedures. You may also be required to identify common medications and their affect on the exercise response (see ACSM, 2000; appendix A). In chapter 15, we provide additional practice questions directly relating to this KSA category, written in the form of case studies.

PRACTICE QUESTIONS

Instructions: Each question is followed by either four or five possible answers. Select the *best* answer to the question.

____ 1. Mr. Smith is a 39-year-old smoker who maintains an active life-style. Information obtained from a medical history and physical examination revealed the following: BP = 141/91; total serum cholesterol = 180; high-density lipoprotein = 61; mother died of a heart attack at 64 years of age. What is Mr. Smith's initial risk stratification?

    a. low risk

     b. moderate risk

     c. high risk

     d. grave risk

____ 2. What should an informed consent form include?

     a. an explanation of the tests to be administered, possible risks and discomforts, possible medications the participant may and may not take prior to exercise testing, freedom of consent, and signatures of both the participant and a witness

     b. an explanation of the test to be administered, possible risks and discomforts, benefits to be expected, freedom of consent, and signature of the participant

     c. an explanation of the tests to be administered, possible risks and discomforts, benefits to be expected, freedom of consent, and signatures of both the participant and a witness

     d. an explanation of the tests to be administered, possible risks and discomforts, the participant's responsibilities, benefits to be expected, inquiries, freedom of consent, and signatures of both the participant and a witness

     e. None of the above answers contain all of the important elements needed in an informed consent form.

____ 3. Which statement is true regarding informed consent?

     a. It should be obtained before an exercise test and before participation in a supervised exercise program.

     b. It should be obtained before an exercise test but is not needed prior to a supervised exercise program.

     c. It should be sent to the potential exercise participant, and the signed form should be mailed to the exercise program director one week prior to program participation.

     d. It should include an explanation of medications the participant should take to reduce muscle soreness.

____ 4. Of the following, which is not an objective of a CR fitness assessment in a low-risk individual?

     a. provide bases for the development of an exercise prescription

     b. to motivate one to begin an exercise program

c. to identify CV disease

d. *b* and *c*

e. *a*, *b*, and *c*

_____ 5. Which of the following represents a rank order of the most accurate technique to the least accurate technique for determining body composition?

    a. hydrostatic, skinfold, anthropometric, bioelectrical impedance, infrared interactance

    b. hydrostatic, anthropometric, skinfold, infrared interactance, bioelectrical impedance

    c. hydrostatic, skinfold, anthropometric, infrared interactance, bioelectrical impedance

    d. infrared interactance, skinfold, bioelectrical impedance, anthropometric, hydrostatic

    e. bioelectrical impedance, skinfold hydrostatic, anthropometric, infrared interactance

_____ 6. Of the following tests, which one relies on HR recovery as an indicator of cardiorespiratory fitness?

    a. YMCA submaximal cycle ergometry protocol

    b. YMCA three-minute step test

    c. Harvard step test

    d. Rockport one-mile fitness walk

_____ 7. Barring complications, a submaximal treadmill exercise test is often terminated when the client obtains a predetermined HR endpoint of what percentage of age predicted maximal HR?

    a. 55

    b. 65

    c. 75

    d. 85

    e. 95

_____ 8. Of the five Korotkoff sounds (phases), which is considered to represent SBP in adults?

    a. 1

    b. 2

    c. 3

    d. 4

    e. 5

___ 9. As an exercise professional, what should you direct a low-risk male, interested in beginning a low- to moderate-intensity exercise program, to do first?

    a. receive a physician's clearance

    b. contact a cardiologist to take a GXT

    c. take the Physical Activity Readiness Questionnaire

    d. take the Cooper 12-minute run test

___ 10. Which of the following individuals should receive medical clearance before participating in a vigorous exercise program?

    a. a 28-year-old male with one CAD risk factor (no signs or symptoms)

    b. a 28-year-old female with one CAD risk factor (no signs or symptoms)

    c. a 46-year-old male (no signs or symptoms)

    d. a 46-year-old female (no signs or symptoms)

    e. None of these individuals needs prior medical clearance.

___ 11. Of the following, which is not an absolute contraindication to exercise testing?

    a. acute infection

    b. uncontrolled metabolic disease

    c. uncontrolled atrial arrhythmia

    d. unstable angina

___ 12. An examination of Ms. Johnson's medical file reveals the following significant facts: complicated pregnancy, unstable angina, and uncontrolled diabetes. Which of these facts, if any, represents an absolute contraindication to exercise testing?

    a. complicated pregnancy

    b. unstable angina

    c. unstable angina and uncontrolled diabetes

    d. None of these is an absolute contraindication to exercise testing.

___ 13. Which laboratory tests should be obtained before an exercise test for an individual classified as apparently healthy (low risk)?

    a. chest X ray

    b. 12-lead resting ECG

    c. pulmonary function test

    d. total serum cholesterol

    e. *b* and *d*

___ 14. Which of the following statements is true regarding the limitations of an informed consent form?

    a. A signed informed consent form offers no legal protection and therefore should not be incorporated in an exercise program.

    b. All informed consent forms should be reviewed by local legal counsel before implementation.

    c. After signing an informed consent form, it is still possible for the professional to be sued.

    d. There are no limitations; once participants have signed the informed consent form, they have forfeited their right to sue.

    e. *b* and *c*

___ 15. For how many hours preceding physical fitness testing should the participant be instructed to avoid food, tobacco, alcohol, and caffeine?

    a. two

    b. three

    c. five

    d. eight

___ 16. What is considered the gold standard for determining body composition?

    a. bioelectrical impedance analysis

    b. hydrostatic weighing

    c. infrared interactance

    d. skinfold measurements

___ 17. Which of the following best describes the appropriate abdominal skinfold site?

    a. horizontal fold taken two centimeters to the left of the umbilicus

    b. vertical fold taken two centimeters to the right of the umbilicus

    c. horizontal fold taken four centimeters to the left of the umbilicus

    d. vertical fold taken four centimeters to the right of the umbilicus

___ 18. Which of the following best describes the appropriate medial calf skinfold site?

    a. horizontal fold taken two centimeters from the midline of the medial border

    b. vertical fold taken two centimeters from the midline of the medial border

    c. horizontal fold taken on the midline of the medial border at a level with the calf's greatest circumference

    d. vertical fold taken on the midline of the medial border at a level with the calf's greatest circumference

___ 19. Which of the following best describes the appropriate procedure for obtaining a skinfold measurement?

    a. Measure right side, place caliper three centimeters from thumb and finger, and wait three to four seconds before reading caliper.

    b. Measure left side, place caliper two centimeters from thumb and finger, and wait one to two seconds before reading caliper.

    c. Measure right side, place caliper one centimeter from thumb and finger, and wait one to two seconds before reading caliper.

    d. Measure left side, place caliper one centimeter from thumb and finger, and wait one to two seconds before reading caliper.

___ 20. What is a limitation of using bioelectrical impedance analysis?

    a. It overestimates percentage of body fat in very lean individuals.

b. It underestimates percentage of body fat in men.

c. It underestimates percentage of body fat in very tall individuals (over 6 feet 4 inches).

d. It underestimates percentage of body fat in very short individuals (under 5 feet).

e. One must control client's hydration prior to testing.

_____ 21. Which of the following is required by the YMCA cycle ergometry protocol?

a. one steady state HR measurement between 90 and 110 beats per minute

b. one steady state HR measurement between 110 and 150 beats per minute

c. two steady state HR measurements between 90 and 110 beats per minute

d. two steady state HR measurements between 110 and 150 beats per minute

_____ 22. What should be considered in the selection of an exercise test protocol for an older adult?

a. A cycle ergometer may be preferable to a treadmill.

b. starting the test at a low intensity level of between two and three METs

c. increasing the expected exercise time to 18 to 20 minutes because of the lower starting intensity

d. *a* and *b*

e. *b* and *c*

_____ 23. Barring an abnormal exercise recovery response, all observations (HR, BP, RPE, signs and symptoms) should continue for at least how many minutes after a submaximal cycle ergometer exercise test?

a. two

b. four

c. six

d. eight

___ 24. At what times during a submaximal cycle ergometer exercise test utilizing three-minute stages should BP be monitored?

a. first portion of each minute

b. last portion of each minute

c. first portion of each stage

d. latter portion of each stage

___ 25. What minimal baseline measures should be obtained prior to the start of an exercise test for a low-risk individual?

a. resting HR

b. resting BP

c. resting ECG

d. *a* and *b*

e. *b* and *c*

___ 26. When BP is being measured, the cuff should be deflated at what rate of mmHg per second?

a. 1

b. 2 to 3

c. 5 to 6

d. 7 to 8

___ 27. When BP is being measured, the cuff should be quickly inflated how many mmHg above the SBP?

a. 10

b. 20

c. 30

d. 40

e. 50

___ 28. Which of the following correctly describes the procedure for calibrating a Monark cycle ergometer?

a. Place the cycle on a level surface, attach a 0.5-kilogram weight to the flywheel's belt and spring, pedal at a rate of 50 revolutions per minute, and note whether the pendulum moves to the 0.5-kilogram mark.

b. Place the cycle on a 0.5 percent incline, attach a 0.5-kilogram weight to the flywheel's spring, pedal at a rate of

50 revolutions per minute, and note whether the pendulum moves to the 0.5-kilogram mark.

c. Place the cycle on a level surface, disconnect the flywheel belt, attach a 0.5-kilogram weight to the flywheel's spring, and note whether the pendulum moves to the 0.5-kilogram mark.

d. Place the cycle on a level surface, disconnect the fly-wheel belt, attach a 0.5-kilogram weight to the flywheel's spring, pedal at a rate of 50 revolutions per minute, and note whether the pendulum moves to the 0.5-kilogram mark.

___ 29. Which of the following BP responses would represent a general indication to discontinue a GXT in an apparently healthy adult?

a. SBP drops 20 mmHg with an increase in exercise intensity.

b. SBP rises to 240 mmHg.

c. DBP fails to increase with an increase in exercise intensity.

d. *a* and *c*

___ 30. General indications for discontinuing a GXT in low-risk adults would include all but which of the following?

a. Subject asks to stop test.

b. Subject's HR increases to 170 beats per minute.

c. Subject shows manifestations of severe fatigue.

d. Subject's HR fails to increase with an increase in exercise intensity.

___ 31. Mr. Orr has a BMI of 25.3. This measure indicates that Mr. Orr is

a. underweight

b. normal weight

c. overweight

d. obese

___ 32. Which of the following is a nitrate or nitroglycerin?

a. isosorbide dinitrate (Isordil)

b. nifedipine (Procardia)

    c. bumetanide (Bumex)

    d. propranolol (Inderal)

___ 33. Which of the following is (are) antianginal calcium channel blocker(s)?

    a. propranolol (Inderal)

    b. nifedipine (Procardia)

    c. diltiazem (Cardizem)

    d. *a* and *b*

    e. *b* and *c*

___ 34. Which of the following is an antianginal beta blocker?

    a. furosemide (Lasix)

    b. metoprolol (Lopressor)

    c. ephedrine (Adrenalin)

    d. quinidine (Quinidex)

___ 35. Which of the following is a diuretic?

    a. furosemide (Lasix)

    b. captopril (Capoten)

    c. quinapril (Accupril)

    d. diltiazem (Cardizem)

___ 36. Which of the following is known as an angiotensin-converting enzyme inhibitor?

    a. propranolol (Inderal)

    b. metoprolol (Lopressor)

    c. furosemide (Lasix)

    d. captopril (Capoten)

___ 37. Which of the following is a peripheral vasodilator?

    a. acebutolol (Sectral)

    b. hydralazine (Apresoline)

    c. metoprolol (Lopressor)

    d. prazosin (Minipress)

___ 38. Which of the following selections, if any, is an (are) antiar-rhythmic medication(s)?

    a. quinidine (Quinidex)

    b. tocainide (Tonocard)

    c. disopyramide (Norpace)

    d. *a, b,* and *c*

    e. none of these

___ 39. Which of the following, if any, is (are) bronchodilator(s)?

    a. albuterol (Bronkosol)

    b. epinephrine (alupent)

    c. *a* and *b*

    d. none of these

___ 40. How may the ingestion of nicotine influence one's response to exercise?

    a. by increasing both SBP and DBP, decreasing HR, and increasing pulse pressure

    b. by increasing SBP, decreasing DBP, increasing HR, and decreasing pulse pressure

    c. by increasing SBP, DBP, and HR

    d. by increasing SBP, decreasing DBP, increasing HR, and increasing pulse pressure

___ 41. How may the ingestion of an antihistamine influence one's response to exercise?

    a. no effect on BP but an increase in HR and exercise capacity

    b. no effect on HR but an increase in BP and exercise capacity

    c. no effect on HR or BP but an increase in exercise capacity

    d. no effect on HR, BP, ECG, or exercise capacity

___ 42. What effect may the ingestion of alcohol have on one's response to exercise?

    a. It increases exercise capacity.

    b. It may provoke arrhythmias.

    c. It decreases HR.

    d. It decreases both HR and BP.

___ 43. How may the ingestion of caffeine influence one's response to exercise?

     a. It may provoke arrhythmias.

     b. It may provoke increase in HR and BP in a caffeine-naive user.

     c. It provokes little to no change in HR or BP in the frequent caffeine user.

     d. *b* and *c*

     e. *a*, *b*, and *c*

___ 44. How may the ingestion of diet pills containing sympathomimetic amines influence one's response to exercise?

     a. It increases HR and BP.

     b. It increases HR but decreases BP.

     c. It significantly improves sprinting speed.

     d. *a* and *c*

     e. *b* and *c*

___ 45. What is the influence of ingesting minor tranquilizers on one's response to exercise?

     a. no significant effect on HR, BP, or exercise capacity except for the side benefit of controlling anxiety

     b. no significant effect on HR or BP except for the side benefit of controlling anxiety and increasing exercise capacity

     c. increase in HR, BP, and exercise capacity

     d. increase in HR and BP but decrease in exercise capacity

REFERENCES FOR FURTHER STUDY

1. ACSM. (2001). *ACSM's resource manual for guidelines for exercise testing and prescription* (4th ed.). Philadelphia: Lippincott Williams & Wilkins.

2. ACSM. (2000). *ACSM's guidelines for exercise testing and prescription* (6th ed.). Philadelphia: Lippincott Williams & Wilkins.

3. Howley, E.T., & Franks, B.D. (2003). *Health fitness instructor's handbook* (4th ed.). Champaign, IL: Human Kinetics.

ANSWERS

Question number	Answer	KSA number	Reference	Page number
1	b	2.6.0.1	2	24
2	d	2.6.0.5	2	53
3	a	2.6.0.5	2	51
4	c	1.6.1	1	361
5	a	2.6.0.13	2	59-68
6	c	2.6.0.8	1	363
7	d	2.6.0.15	2	74
8	a	2.6.0.9	2	40
9	c	2.6.0.2	2	23
10	c	2.6.0.2	2	27
11	b	2.6.0.3	2	50
12	b	2.6.0.3	2	50
13	d	2.6.0.5	2	38
14	e	2.6.0.4	1	626-631
15	b	2.6.0.7	2	58
16	b	2.6.0.12	2	60
17	b	2.6.0.10	2	65
18	d	2.6.0.10	2	65
19	c	2.6.0.10	2	65
20	e	2.6.0.12	1	395
21	d	2.6.0.8	2	75
22	d	2.6.0.16	2	225
23	b	2.6.0.6	2	72

Question number	Answer	KSA number	Reference	Page number
24	d	2.6.0.6	2	72
25	d	2.6.0.6	2	77
26	b	2.6.0.9	2	40
27	b	2.6.0.9	2	40
28	c	2.6.0.19	3	92-95
29	a	2.6.0.15	2	80
30	b	2.6.0.15	2	80
31	c	2.6.0.14	2	63
32	a	2.6.0.17.1	2	274
33	e	2.6.0.17.1	2	274
34	b	2.6.0.17.1	2	273
35	a	2.3.0.17.2	2	275
36	d	2.6.0.17.2	2	275
37	b	2.6.0.17.2	2	274
38	d	2.6.0.17.3	2	275-276
39	c	2.6.0.17.4	2	276
40	c	2.6.0.18	2	281
41	d	2.6.0.18	2	281
42	b	2.6.0.18	2	281
43	e	2.6.0.18	2	282
44	a	2.6.0.18	2	282
45	a	2.6.0.18	2	280

Safety, Injury Prevention, and Emergency Care

This chapter contains 33 practice questions to help you study for the 16 objectives listed under the ACSM certification KSAs in the category Safety, Injury Prevention, and Emergency Care. Pay close attention to the "skill" objectives, as you may be tested on this information in your practical exam. On the basis of previous ACSM Health/Fitness Instructor certification examinations, you will receive approximately five questions from this category.

Before taking the certification exam, you must provide documentation showing that you have successfully completed a CPR course. We also recommend taking a standard first aid course. The CPR and first aid training, review of those course materials, and correctly answering the questions contained within this chapter will adequately prepare you to take this portion of the certification examination.

PRACTICE QUESTIONS

Instructions: Each question is followed by either four or five possible answers. Select the *best* answer to the question.

_____ 1. Which of the following are essential to all emergency medical plans?

    a. All personnel involved with exercise testing should have CPR certification.

    b. At least one ACLS certified person should be on board.

    c. At least one paramedic should be on board.

    d. *a* and *b*

    e. *a*, *b*, and *c*

____ 2. What is the correct order of events to find the correct hand position for the adult in CPR?

    a. Use the heel of your hand to apply pressure on the sternum; find the lower edge of the victim's rib cage; place the heel of one hand on the sternum next to your index finger and place your other hand on top of it; slide your middle and index fingers up to the edge of the rib cage to the notch where the ribs meet the sternum; place your middle and index fingers on the notch where the ribs meet the sternum.

    b. Find the lower edge of the victim's rib cage, place the heel of one hand on the sternum next to your index finger and place your other hand on top of it; use the heel of your hand to apply pressure on the sternum; slide your middle and index fingers up the edge of the rib cage to the notch where the ribs meet the sternum; place your middle and index fingers on the notch where the ribs meet the sternum.

    c. Find the lower edge of the victim's rib cage; slide your middle and index fingers up the edge of the rib cage to the notch where the ribs meet the sternum; place the heel of one hand on the sternum next to your index finger and place your other hand on top of it; place your middle and index fingers on the notch where the ribs meet the sternum; use the heel of your hand to apply pressure on the sternum.

    d. Find the lower edge of the victim's rib cage; slide your middle and index fingers up the edge of the rib cage to the notch where the ribs meet the sternum; place your middle and index fingers on the notch where the ribs meet the sternum; place the heel of one hand on the sternum next to your index finger and place your other hand on top of it; use the heel of your hand to apply pressure on the sternum.

____ 3. All personnel must know what about the facility's emergency plan?

    a. that emergency plans should be posted

    b. the location of the telephone and emergency number

    c. the location of all emergency equipment

d. *a* and *b*

e. *a*, *b*, and *c*

____ 4. At a facility such as a YMCA, a pool, or a local community park without emergency equipment, what is the responsibility of the first rescuer in a potentially life-threatening situation?

a. to instruct victim to stop activity

b. to remain with victim until symptoms subside

c. to call the EMS

d. *a* and *b*

e. *a*, *b*, and *c*

____ 5. At a gym or exercise facility with basic emergency equipment (e.g., a defibrillator or drugs), what is the responsibility of the second rescuer on the scene in a life-threatening situation?

a. to call the EMS

b. to wait and direct the emergency team

c. to assist first rescuer and bring blood pressure cuff and ECG monitor to site

d. *a* and *b*

e. *a*, *b*, and *c*

____ 6. What is the first-aid procedure for bleeding?

a. Cover the wound with a clean dressing and press firmly against the wound with the hand.

b. Immobilize area with a splint.

c. Apply a tourniquet when the bleeding is serious.

d. *a* and *b*

e. *a*, *b*, and *c*

____ 7. What should be done if a person experiences dizziness or syncope?

a. Place the individual on his/her side.

b. Give the individual some form of sugar, preferably in liquid form.

c. Position the individual on his/her back and elevate the legs 8 to 10 inches (only if there is no suspected head or back injury).

    d. Restrain the individual and place a bit block between the teeth.

___ 8. First aid for dyspnea includes

    a. giving the individual oral insulin

    b. using an AED immediately and activating EMS

    c. maintaining an open airway and activating EMS if symptoms are not relieved

    d. placing the victim on his/her side in case there is vomiting

___ 9. First aid for heat exhaustion includes all but which of the following?

    a. removing the victim from the sun to a ventilated and cooler area

    b. placing the victim in shock position (supine and feet elevated)

    c. transporting the victim to the hospital immediately

    d. *a* and *b*

    e. *a, b,* and *c*

___ 10. To ensure participant safety in a group exercise setting,

    a. develop guidelines and proper protocol for an emergency during an exercise session

    b. develop guidelines for the institution for emergency drills

    c. have an ACLS certified individual at each exercise session

    d. *a* and *b*

    e. *a, b,* and *c*

___ 11. To ensure participant safety in a group exercise setting,

    a. conduct a preparticipation health appraisal to determine individuals who may require additional medical evaluation

    b. require all participants to receive approval to exercise from their physicians

    c. only include participants who are between the ages of 21 and 35 years

    d. *a* and *b*

    e. *a, b,* and *c*

___ 12. Musculoskeletal injury increases exponentially with what type of training?

    a. running with high training errors

    b. running with a high volume and frequency

    c. running 30 minutes a day, three times a week

    d. *a* and *b*

    e. *a*, *b*, and *c*

___ 13. What is (are) the potential cause(s) of overuse injuries?

    a. repeated microtrauma

    b. fatigue

    c. running down hills

    d. *a* and *b*

    e. *a*, *b*, and *c*

___ 14. Training at high altitude could result in which of the following responses?

    a. an increase in $\dot{V}O_2$max upon return to sea level

    b. inability to train at an optimal workload to improve fitness level

    c. polycythemia

    d. *a* and *b*

    e. *a*, *b*, and *c*

___ 15. Exercising in a polluted environment may result in

    a. irritation of the airways leading to bronchoconstriction

    b. reduction of alveolar diffusion capacity

    c. reduction of oxygen transport capacity

    d. *a* and *b*

    e. *a*, *b*, and *c*

___ 16. A 65-year-old male is working out in the fitness facility on a bicycle ergometer. He begins to feel light-headed and nauseated. His speech is slurred. He collapses. You are on the exercise floor and observe this situation. What should you do first?

    a. Make sure the victim is lying down and check the airway and circulation.

    b. Call the EMS.

    c. Call the EMS and go to the entrance and wait for the ambulance.

    d. Give CPR immediately.

___ 17. You are helping out with an exercise test on a 50-year-old female with moderate valvular heart disease. During the test, she complains of uncomfortable chest pain (3.0 on the angina scale). It is the decision of the physician to stop the test. What should you do?

    a. Assist the physician and the exercise physiologist/clinical exercise specialist.

    b. Bring all the emergency equipment to the area.

    c. Call the EMS.

    d. *a* and *b*

    e. *a*, *b*, and *c*

___ 18. You are supervising the running track where participants are walking and jogging. One of the walkers wanders from his designated walking lane into the path of a jogger absorbed in conversation. The walker is accidentally pushed to the floor of the track. What should you do?

    a. Remain with the victim until injury symptoms subside.

    b. Use basic first aid (if necessary).

    c. Call EMS immediately and send someone to the entrance to wait.

    d. *a* and *b*

    e. *a*, *b*, and *c*

___ 19. Chronic low back pain is associated with

    a. reduced mobility in trunk flexion

    b. reduced mobility in lateral flexion and extension of trunk

    c. decreased straight-leg raising

    d. *a* and *b*

    e. *a*, *b*, and *c*

___ 20. Which of the following exercises is (are) recommended for low back pain?

    a. aerobic exercise

    b. cat stretch

    c. straight-leg sit-ups

    d. *a* and *b*

    e. *a*, *b*, and *c*

___ 21. Straight-leg sit-ups are not recommended because

    a. the low back hyperextends caused by use of the hip flexors

    b. high compressional forces are placed on the spinal discs; cervical ligaments can be damaged

    c. overstretching of the lumbar ligament may occur

    d. *a* and *b*

    e. *a*, *b*, and *c*

___ 22. The plough is not a recommended exercise because

    a. those with osteoporosis or arthritis are at particular risk

    b. spinal discs could be damaged

    c. damage may occur to the medical collateral ligament

    d. *a* and *b*

    e. *a*, *b*, and *c*

___ 23. For the exercise professional, being accused of failure to respond adequately to an untoward event with appropriate emergency care is a claim that would most likely result in which one of the following?

    a. participant withdrawal from the fitness program

    b. litigation procedures against the Health/Fitness Instructor or the facility

    c. loss of employment for the Health/Fitness Instructor

    d. an increase in liability insurance for the Health/Fitness Instructor

____ 24. In a fitness facility, it is the employer's responsibility to have documented guidelines on emergency procedures and properly communicate these to all employees. What is the responsibility of the Health/Fitness Instructor?

    a. to evaluate and render a diagnosis of a medical condition or accident once appropriate training has been obtained

    b. to make sure that emergency training is obtained and updated to prevent careless performance in an emergency situation

    c. to assign someone to carry out emergency care according to the instructions in the facility legal document

    d. *a* and *b*

    e. *a*, *b*, and *c*

____ 25. For the instructor to be protected from liability in all emergency-response situations, what must the employer (facility) do?

    a. Communicate the emergency medical procedures to the instructor.

    b. Provide for appropriate training and updates.

    c. Put the emergency plan into action with periodic drills (at least twice per year).

    d. *a* and *b*

    e. *a*, *b*, and *c*

____ 26. Which of the following matches the musculoskeletal injury to its description?

    a. contusion: slight bleeding into tissues while the skin remains unbroken

    b. sprain: tearing of a muscle or tendon

    c. strain: tearing of ligamentous tissue

    d. fracture: displacement of a particular bone from its normal position

____ 27. Cardiovascular/pulmonary complications can include which of the following?

    a. tachycardia: myocardial contraction rate of more than 100 beats per minute; bradycardia: myocardial contraction rate of less than 60

b. hypotension: a condition in which BP is inadequate for normal perfusion and oxygenation of the tissues; hypertension: a major risk factor for CAD, stroke, congestive heart failure, and chronic renal failure

c. hypoventilation: a pulmonary ventilation rate that is metabolically necessary for exchange pulmonary gases; tachypnea: an abnormally rapid rate of breathing as seen in fever

d. *a* and *b*

e. *a*, *b*, and *c*

___ 28. Which of the following correctly matches the metabolic abnormalities to the corresponding descriptions?

a. hyperthermia: body temperature below normal; hypothermia: low body temperature due to exposure to cold temperature

b. fainting: a loss of consciousness; syncope: a brief lapse in consciousness caused by a decrease in O_2 to the brain

c. hyperglycemia: a less-than-normal amount of glucose in the blood caused by administration of too much insulin; hypoglycemia: a greater-than-normal amount of glucose in the blood

d. *a* and *b*

e. *a*, *b*, and *c*

___ 29. What immediate care is appropriate for most open wounds?

a. application of direct pressure over the site to stop bleeding

b. application of a sterile dressing to protect the wound from contamination

c. maintenance of an open airway

d. *a* and *b*

e. *a*, *b*, and *c*

___ 30. For injuries to the muscle and joints, appropriate first-aid care would include which of the following?

a. stopping activity and keeping the victim from applying any weight-bearing to the affected limb

b. the use of a blanket-type splint for the foot and elevation of the limb

c. the application of ice and compression to the injury

d. *a* and *b*

e. *a*, *b*, and *c*

___ 31. A 12-year-old female started coughing and wheezing, unable to catch her breath, while running on an indoor track. What immediate first aid is appropriate?

a. maintaining an open airway

b. administering or helping the girl administer her oral bronchodilator medication

c. rushing her to the hospital

d. *a* and *b*

e. *a*, *b*, and *c*

___ 32. A preventive maintenance/repair program for weight-training equipment would involve which of the following procedures?

a. daily: clean upholstery with a mild soap and water solution

b. weekly: use a vinyl upholstery protectant on all equipment

c. monthly: inspect cables, nuts, and bolts of all weight machines utilizing such devices

d. *a* and *b*

e. *a*, *b*, and *c*

___ 33. A cardiovascular equipment preventive maintenance/repair schedule would include which of the following daily procedures?

a. cleaning monorail of the rower machines, washing the seat of the rower with a mild soap and water solution

b. cleaning the seat and frame of the bicycle ergometer with a mild soap and water solution

c. inspecting the housing, belts, and electronic components on each of the stair climbers

d. *a* and *b*

e. *a*, *b*, and *c*

REFERENCES FOR FURTHER STUDY

1. ACSM. (2001). *ACSM's resource manual for guidelines for exercise testing and prescription* (4th ed.). Philadelphia: Lippincott Williams & Wilkins.
2. ACSM. (2000). *ACSM's guidelines for exercise testing and prescription* (6th ed.). Philadelphia: Lippincott Williams & Wilkins.

ANSWERS

Question number	Answer	KSA number	Reference	Page number
1	d	1.7.0	2	283
2	d	1.7.0	1	103
3	e	1.7.1	2	283
			1	633, 650
4	d	1.7.1	2	288
5	d	1.7.1	2	291
6	a	1.7.2	1	656
7	c	1.7.2	1	656
8	c	1.7.2	1	656
9	d	1.7.2	1	656
10	d	1.7.3	1	650
11	a	1.7.3	1	355
12	d	1.7.4	1	492
13	e	1.7.4	1	493
14	b	1.7.5	1	218
15	e	1.7.5	1	220
16	a	2.7.0	2	288
17	e	2.7.0	2	289

Question number	Answer	KSA number	Reference	Page number
18	d	2.7.0	2	286
19	e	1.7.7	1	384
20	d	1.7.7	1	124
21	b	1.7.8	1	659
22	d	1.7.8	1	659
23	b	2.7.3	1	629
24	b	2.7.3	2	283
25	e	2.7.3	2	283
			1	630
26	a	2.7.4	1	655
27	d	2.7.4	1	501
28	b	2.7.4	1	657
29	d	2.7.5	1	655, 666
30	e	2.7.5	1	656, 657
31	d	2.7.5	1	332, 509
32	e	2.7.6	1	643, 645
33	d	2.7.6	1	643

11

Exercise Programming

Of the 10 ACSM KSA categories, Exercise Programming is the most comprehensive. When studying, be sure you understand each component of the objective before moving on to the next objective. A fair number of the KSAs in this category refer to your ability to "teach" and/or "demonstrate" specific exercises or exercise modifications. As such, these KSAs may not be assessed in the written portion of this certification examination but, instead, in the practical portion of the examination. Additionally, questions related to metabolic equations and exercise programming skills have not been addressed at length in this chapter. Instead, we have provided a separate chapter on each (chapter 14, *Solving Metabolic Equations* and chapter 15, *Analyzing Case Studies*) in order to better prepare you for this important aspect of the certification examination. Based on previous ACSM Health/Fitness Instructor certification examinations, you are likely to receive approximately 22 questions from this category.

PRACTICE QUESTIONS

Instructions: Each question is followed by either four or five possible answers. Select the *best* answer to the question.

_____ 1. What mode of prolonged exercise is most likely to produce significant improvement in maximal aerobic capacity?

　　a. rhythmic small-muscle activity

　　b. rhythmic large-muscle activity

   c. nonrhythmic small-muscle activity

   d. nonrhythmic large-muscle activity

_____ 2. What intensity of exercise is needed to develop CRF in an apparently healthy individual?

   a. 30/40 to 50 percent of maximum HR

   b. 55/65 to 90 percent of maximum HR

   c. 40/50 to 85 percent of HRR

   d. *a* and *c*

   e. *b* and *c*

_____ 3. What does the ACSM recommend regarding the duration of exercise for the development of CRF?

   a. high-intensity (>90 percent) exercise for 5 to 10 minutes

   b. multiple 10-minute exercise sessions for the severely deconditioned

   c. continuous aerobic activity for 20 to 60 minutes

   d. *a* and *b*

   e. *b* and *c*

_____ 4. What does the ACSM recommend regarding the frequency of cardiorespiratory exercise?

   a. one to two sessions per week for individuals who possess a 3 to 5 MET capacity

   b. one to two sessions per day for individuals who possess a capacity >5 METs

   c. three to five sessions per day for individuals who possess a capacity >5 METs

   d. three to five sessions per week for individuals who possess a capacity >5 METs

_____ 5. Which statement best describes the movement known as "exercise lite"?

   a. Every adult should accumulate 15 minutes or more of moderate-intensity physical activity over the course of most days.

   b. Every adult should accumulate 15 minutes or more of high-intensity physical activity over the course of most days.

    c. Every adult should accumulate 30 minutes or more of moderate-intensity physical activity over the course of most days.

    d. Every adult should accumulate 30 minutes or more of high-intensity physical activity over the course of most days.

_____ 6. Placing a muscle or muscle group under a stress greater than it is accustomed to handling is an example of what principle?

    a. overload

    b. specificity

    c. isotonic resistance

    d. isokinetic resistance

_____ 7. Select the term(s) that best represent(s) the following: using high-intensity, low-volume resistance training for the development of muscular strength, as well as using low-intensity, high-volume resistance training for the development of muscular endurance.

    a. overload principle

    b. progressive resistance

    c. principle of specificity

    d. *a* and *b*

_____ 8. A music tempo of approximately how many beats per minute is appropriate for the warm-up phase of an aerobic exercise class?

    a. 100

    b. 125

    c. 140

    d. 160

_____ 9. Which of the following exercises could be considered a safer alternative exercise for the plough?

    a. 90-degree squat

    b. double knee to chest

    c. supine crunch

    d. standing hamstring stretch

_____10. Which of the following exercises could be considered a safer alternative exercise for the standing toe touch?

    a. standing hamstring stretch

    b. hurdler's stretch

    c. seated hamstring stretch

    d. both *b* and *c*

_____11. Which of the following exercises could be considered a safer alternative exercise for the traditional hurdler's stretch?

    a. seated hamstring stretch

    b. double knee to chest

    c. standing toe touch

    d. plough

_____12. For individuals not acclimated to temperatures greater than 24 °C, one would expect heart rate to increase how many beats per minute with each degree increase in temperature?

    a. 1

    b. 2

    c. 3

    d. 4

_____13. What should be incorporated with warm-up exercises performed before sport participation?

    a. a general warm-up followed by a sport-specific warm-up

    b. a sport-specific warm-up followed by a general warm-up

    c. only a general warm-up

    d. only a sport-specific warm-up

_____14. Which of the following is *not* a value of a cool-down period following an exercise session?

    a. It aids in the removal of by-products of strenuous exercise.

    b. It aids in the prevention of venous pooling in the legs.

    c. It reduces the risk of injury.

    d. It allows the circulatory system to return gradually to a resting state.

____15. How does a structured warm-up before an exercise session prepare the body for additional intense activity?

    a. It increases muscle blood flow and temperature.

    b. It increases connective tissue elasticity.

    c. It increases muscle viscosity.

    d. *a* and *b*

    e. *b* and *c*

____16. What is the proper exercise sequence for the following activities?

    a. slow jog, static stretching, two-mile run, quarter-mile walk, static stretching

    b. slow jog, two-mile run, quarter-mile walk

    c. two-mile run, quarter-mile walk, static stretching

    d. slow jog, dynamic stretching, two-mile run, quarter-mile walk, dynamic stretching

____17. Which term best describes a type of muscular action that acts as a braking force and involves muscle elongation during tension development?

    a. concentric

    b. isometric

    c. eccentric

    d. isotonic

____18. Which of the following is (are) *incorrect* regarding the nature of an eccentric muscle action?

    a. muscle elongation during force production

    b. maximum effort not great enough to overcome an external force applied in an opposing direction

    c. a braking force to control speed of movement

    d. less muscle soreness compared to that from a concentric contraction

    e. *b* and *d*

____19. What term best describes a type of muscle action in which the muscle shortens, causing movement at a joint?

    a. concentric

    b. eccentric

c. isometric

d. plyometric

_____20. What term best describes a type of muscle action in which there is no joint movement and no change in the length of the agonist muscle?

a. concentric

b. eccentric

c. isometric

d. isotonic

_____21. Which term best describes a type of muscle action in which the speed of muscle contraction is precisely controlled?

a. isokinetic

b. isometric

c. isotonic

d. plyometric

_____22. What is the Valsalva maneuver?

a. rapidly exhaling during a maximal muscular contraction

b. rapidly inhaling during a maximal muscular contraction

c. rapidly exhaling during a submaximal muscular contraction

d. breath-holding with a closed glottis

_____23. Regarding the Valsalva maneuver, which of the following statements is *incorrect?*

a. It causes an increase in abdominal cavity pressure.

b. It causes an increase in thoracic cavity pressure.

c. It can cause an acute increase in both SBP and DBP.

d. It facilitates the return of blood to the heart.

_____24. What term best describes a type of muscle action in which the prime mover exerts force greater than resistance, resulting in muscle shortening and joint movement?

a. isometric

b. isokinetic

c. isotonic

d. plyometric

____25. Which term refers to a reduction in the size of a muscle or body part?

    a. accretion

    b. atrophy

    c. hyperplasia

    d. hypertrophy

____26. Which term refers to an increase in the size of a muscle or other body part caused by cell enlargement?

    a. accretion

    b. atrophy

    c. hyperplasia

    d. hypertrophy

____27. Which term refers to the eccentric loading of a muscle just before concentric muscular contraction?

    a. isometric

    b. isotonic

    c. isokinetic

    d. plyometric

____28. What is quantified by the RPE scale?

    a. degree of difficulty in breathing during exercise

    b. degree of chest pain during exercise

    c. degree of light-headedness during exercise

    d. subjective feeling of physical effort during exercise

____29. Using the original RPE scale (6 to 20 points), what level of perceived exertion is associated with a CRF training effect?

    a. 6 to 9 points

    b. 10 to 11 points

    c. 12 to 16 points

    d. none of these

____30. The RPE scale is useful for

    a. determining impending fatigue

    b. determining degree of leg pain

    c. determining degree of breathlessness

    d. none of these

_____31. The RPE scale allows the exerciser to report subjective feelings during exercise taking what into consideration?

    a. general fatigue

    b. environmental conditions

    c. individual fitness level

    d. *a* and *b*

    e. *a*, *b*, and *c*

_____32. What is the predicted maximal HR (beats per minute) for a 37-year-old male?

    a. 153

    b. 163

    c. 173

    d. 183

_____33. Bob is a 42-year-old active nonsmoker who has received physician clearance to take part in a CRF exercise program. According to ACSM guidelines, what is the range of Bob's exercise intensity (beats per minute) based on a percentage of HR max?

    a. 71 to 107

    b. 116 to 160

    c. 110 to 130

    d. 150 to 180

_____34. Beth is a 52-year-old active nonsmoker who has received physician clearance to participate in a CRF exercise program. Beth's resting HR is 72 beats per minute, and during a GXT her HR max was determined to be 168 beats per minute. Based on ACSM guidelines, what would be Beth's exercise intensity (beats per minute) as measured by the HRR method?

    a. 105 to 125

    b. 110 to 130

    c. 120 to 154

    d. 135 to 180

_____35. What is the predicted maximal HR range in beats per minute for 68 percent of the population for individuals who are 27 years of age?

    a. 172 to 192

    b. 181 to 205

    c. 195 to 210

    d. 211 to 220

_____36. Jim's maximum HR is 189 beats per minute, while his resting HR is 62 beats per minute. What would be Jim's target HR range (beats per minute) as calculated by the HRR method?

    a. 126 to 170

    b. 138 to 164

    c. 140 to 180

    d. 149 to 189

_____37. Which of the following is (are) true regarding the RPE scale?

    a. It is unreliable in approximately 30 percent of the population.

    b. It is useful for monitoring exercise intensity in individuals who have difficulty palpating HR.

    c. It is not recommended if the exercise participant's HR response is known to be altered because of a change in medication.

    d. *a* and *b*

    e. *b* and *c*

_____38. When monitoring exercise HR at the carotid artery, how should the participant palpate the carotid artery?

    a. Use the thumb to apply moderate pressure.

    b. Use the index and middle fingers to apply heavy pressure.

    c. Use the thumb and index finger to apply light pressure.

    d. Use the index and middle fingers to apply light pressure.

_____39. When riding a cycle, when the leg is at the bottom of the downstroke, the knee should be bent approximately how many degrees?

    a. 5

    b. 10

c. 15

d. 20

____40. Which of the following exercises is (are) most appropriate for someone with low back pain?

  a. full sit-ups with feet held

  b. double leg raise

  c. pelvic tilt

  d. *a* and *b*

  e. *b* and *c*

____41. How is exercise intensity best monitored during pregnancy?

  a. palpating HR at the radial artery

  b. palpating HR at the brachial artery

  c. using the RPE scale

  d. using a dyspnea scale

____42. During pregnancy, which activity should be avoided after the first trimester?

  a. any exercise in the supine position

  b. any exercise in the prone position

  c. cycling

  d. swimming

____43. What aerobic intensity range and resistance training would be included in an appropriate exercise program for individuals diagnosed with hypertension?

  a. 40 to 70 percent and a resistance-training component consisting of both high repetitions/low resistance and isometric activities

  b. 40 to 70 percent and a resistance-training component consisting of moderate isometric activities

  c. 40 to 70 percent and a resistance-training component consisting of high repetitions and low resistance

  d. 75 to 85 percent and a resistance-training component consisting of low repetitions and high resistance

  e. 80 to 90 percent and a resistance-training component consisting of high repetitions and low resistance

____44. How should the duration of exercise be modified for an obese individual?

    a. Limit duration to 20 minutes.

    b. Keep caloric expenditure to 300 to 500 kcal per session.

    c. Keep caloric expenditure to 500 to 600 kcal per session.

    d. Keep caloric expenditure to 3000 to 3600 kcal per week.

    e. *c* and *d*

____45. Which of the following activities would be most appropriate for an individual who experiences exercise-induced asthma?

    a. brisk walking in cold weather

    b. jogging in cold weather

    c. swimming

    d. *a* and *b*

____46. What are the proper adjustments when one is using the Nautilus® leg extension machine?

    a. Place arms across the chest, adjust seat so that roller pad contacts the middle of the shin, and align knees with axis of machine.

    b. Place arms across the chest, adjust seat so that roller pad contacts shin slightly above the ankles, and align knees with axis of machine.

    c. Grasp handles on each side of seat, align knees with axis of machine, and lean forward as knees are fully extended.

    d. Grasp handles on each side of seat, align knees with axis of machine, and keep back flat against back pad as knees are fully extended.

____47. When spotting the supine dumbbell fly, where should the spotter's hands be positioned?

    a. under or on the performer's elbows

    b. under or on the performer's wrist

    c. on the dumbbells

    d. no spotter needed for this exercise

_____48. Which of the following flexibility exercises is designed to stretch the anterior deltoids and pectoralis major?

    a. behind-the-neck stretch (chicken wing)

    b. pretzel

    c. seated lean-back

    d. plough

_____49. Which form of exercise may be most appropriate for an elderly individual with an impaired gait pattern?

    a. walk on a outdoor track

    b. walk on a indoor treadmill

    c. exercise on a cycle ergometer

    d. exercise on a stair climber

_____50. Which resistance exercise primarily trains the brachialis?

    a. biceps curl

    b. overhead elbow extension

    c. knee flexion

    d. knee extension

_____51. Which of the following best describes the resistance-training system known as an *ascending pyramid?*

    a. performing multiple sets, starting at about 10 to 12 repetitions and systematically increasing resistance over several sets until only one repetition is possible

    b. performing multiple sets starting at 1RM and systematically reducing resistance and increasing repetitions until 10 to 12 repetitions are completed

    c. performing one set of several exercises in succession for the same muscle group, each building upon the other with no rest between exercises

    d. *a* and *b*

    e. none of these

_____52. Performing 12 biceps curls immediately followed by 12 repetitions of triceps extensions is an example of what resistance-training system?

    a. plyometrics

b. pyramiding

c. split routine

d. super sets

_____53. Depth jumping is an example of which of the following?

a. pyramiding

b. plyometrics

c. super sets

d. split routine

_____54. For a person with diabetes, unplanned exercise should be preceded by

a. 5 to 10 grams of extra carbohydrates for every hour of exercise

b. 5 to 10 grams of extra carbohydrates every 30 minutes during exercise

c. 10 to 20 grams of extra carbohydrates for every hour of exercise

d. 10 to 20 grams of extra carbohydrates every 30 minutes of exercise

_____55. A person with diabetes should delay exercise if glucose is greater than

a. 100 mg/dl

b. 150 mg/dl

c. 300 mg/dl without ketones

d. 200 mg/dl without ketones

_____56. Which of the following type of aerobic exercise equipment would be most appropriate for an obese individual?

a. step bench for high-impact aerobics

b. bicycle

c. jump rope

d. treadmill for running

_____57. What is (are) the potential disadvantage(s) of using a stair climber for an aerobic workout?

a. It may aggravate some knee conditions.

b. It requires an element of coordination and balance.

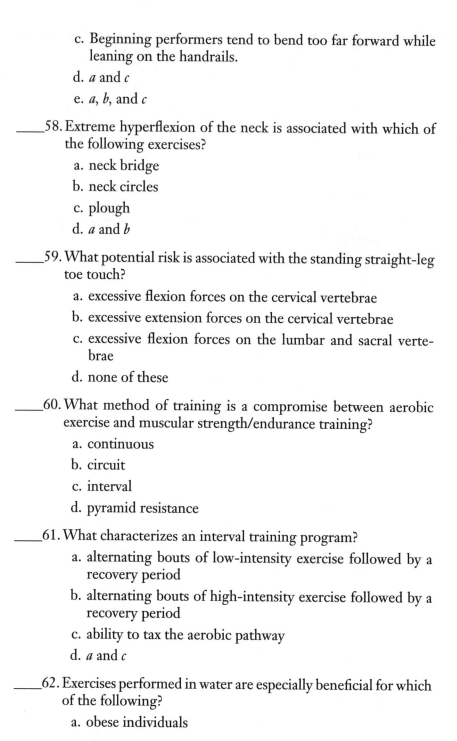

   c. Beginning performers tend to bend too far forward while leaning on the handrails.

   d. *a* and *c*

   e. *a*, *b*, and *c*

_____58. Extreme hyperflexion of the neck is associated with which of the following exercises?

   a. neck bridge

   b. neck circles

   c. plough

   d. *a* and *b*

_____59. What potential risk is associated with the standing straight-leg toe touch?

   a. excessive flexion forces on the cervical vertebrae

   b. excessive extension forces on the cervical vertebrae

   c. excessive flexion forces on the lumbar and sacral vertebrae

   d. none of these

_____60. What method of training is a compromise between aerobic exercise and muscular strength/endurance training?

   a. continuous

   b. circuit

   c. interval

   d. pyramid resistance

_____61. What characterizes an interval training program?

   a. alternating bouts of low-intensity exercise followed by a recovery period

   b. alternating bouts of high-intensity exercise followed by a recovery period

   c. ability to tax the aerobic pathway

   d. *a* and *c*

_____62. Exercises performed in water are especially beneficial for which of the following?

   a. obese individuals

b. pregnant women

c. arthritic patients

d. *a* and *c*

e. *a*, *b*, and *c*

_____63. How can one increase the exercise intensity experienced during water exercise?

    a. by exercising in deeper water

    b. by exercising in shallower water

    c. by jogging in a circle and quickly changing direction, thus being required to jog against the water current

    d. *a* and *c*

    e. *b* and *c*

_____64. Which stretching technique is most likely to require the aid of an exercise partner?

    a. ballistic

    b. dynamic

    c. proprioceptive neuromuscular facilitation

    d. static

_____65. To accommodate different levels of abdominal strength and endurance within the same exercise class, what are the appropriate hand and arm positions for untrained and trained individuals when performing a bent-knee sit-up?

    a. The untrained should place the hands and arms behind the head with elbows bent and fingers interwoven, while the trained should place the hands and arms across the chest.

    b. The untrained should place the hands and arms across the chest, while the trained should position the hands and arms on the thighs.

    c. The untrained should place the hands and arms beside the hips or on the thighs, while the trained should position the hands and arms behind the head, being careful not to hyperflex the neck.

    d. Hand and arm position does not affect the intensity of performing a bent-knee sit-up.

____66. Typical RPE range for acquiring a training effect using the category–ratio scale?

    a. 2 to 3

    b. 4 to 5

    c. 7 to 8

    d. RPE is not used to monitor exercise intensity

REFERENCES FOR FURTHER STUDY

1. ACSM. (2001). *ACSM's resource manual for guidelines for exercise testing and prescription* (4th ed.). Philadelphia: Lippincott Williams & Wilkins.

2. ACSM. (2000). *ACSM's guidelines for exercise testing and prescription* (6th ed.). Philadelphia: Lippincott Williams & Wilkins.

3. Baechle, T.R., & Earle, R.W. (Eds.) (2000). *Essentials of strength training and conditioning (2nd ed.).* Champaign, IL: Human Kinetics.

4. Fleck, S.J., & Kraemer, W.J. (1997). *Designing resistance training programs* (2nd ed.). Champaign, IL: Human Kinetics.

5. Howley, E.T., & Franks, B.D. (2003). *Health fitness instructor's handbook* (4th ed.). Champaign, IL: Human Kinetics.

ANSWERS

Question number	Answer	KSA number	Reference	Page number
1	b	1.8.0	5	167
2	e	1.8.0	2	145
3	e	1.8.0	2	150
4	d	1.8.0	2	151
5	c	1.8.1	5	177
6	a	1.8.3	5	161
7	c	1.8.3	5	162
8	a	1.8.22	5	278
9	b	1.8.25	1	659

Question number	Answer	KSA number	Reference	Page number
10	a	1.8.25	1	659
11	a	1.8.25	1	659
12	a	2.8.0.13	2	18
13	a	1.8.4	5	168
14	c	1.8.5	1	451
15	d	1.8.5	2	141
16	a	1.8.5	5	168
17	c	1.8.6	5	457
18	d	1.8.6	5	457
19	a	1.8.6	5	456
20	c	1.8.6	5	458
21	a	1.8.6	2	83
22	d	1.8.6	5	207
23	d	1.8.6	5	207
24	c	1.8.6	4	18
25	b	1.8.6	5	207
26	d	1.8.6	5	207
27	d	1.8.6	4	35
28	d	1.8.7	1	364
29	c	1.8.7	2	78
30	a	1.8.7	2	79
31	e	1.8.7	2	78
32	d	1.8.9	5	175
33	b	1.8.9	2	145

Question number	Answer	KSA number	Reference	Page number
34	c	1.8.9	2	145
35	b	1.8.9	2	117
36	b	1.8.9	2	147
37	b	1.8.8	2	78-79
38	d	1.8.8	5	416
39	a	1.8.12	2	72
40	c	1.8.10	5	255
41	c	1.8.10	2	231-232
42	a	1.8.10	2	231
43	c	1.8.10	2	208
44	b	1.8.10	2	216
45	c	1.8.10	1	332
46	d	1.8.11	3	376
47	b	1.8.11	3	348
48	c	1.8.13	3	332
49	c	1.8.10	2	225
50	a	1.8.15	3	355
51	a	2.8.0.14	4	124
52	d	2.8.0.14	4	127
53	b	2.8.0.14	5	209-210
54	d	2.8.0.9	2	213
55	c	2.8.0.9	5	325
56	b	2.8.0.19	1	642
57	e	2.8.0.19	1	642

Question number	Answer	KSA number	Reference	Page number
58	c	2.8.0.15	1	659
59	c	2.8.0.15	1	659
60	b	1.8.16	3	152
61	b	1.8.16	3	87
62	e	1.8.21	2	224, 231
63	d	1.8.21	Consult any aquatic exercise text	
64	c	1.8.19	3	325-329
65	c	1.8.20	5	256
66	b	2.8.0.12	2	78

CHAPTER

12

Nutrition and Weight Management

The objectives in this ACSM KSA category, Nutrition and Weight Management, are straightforward, and the readings and references we provide should prepare you adequately for the written examination, even without a special course in nutrition. Note that objectives 2.9.0.5 and 2.9.0.6 require you to demonstrate familiarity with several resource papers. These papers are listed at the end of this chapter in a special Suggested Readings section. We recommend that you obtain these papers and read them carefully. In light of the importance of these readings, we have put less emphasis on practice questions in this chapter. Therefore, you will be able to allot more of your study time for this section of the examination to working through the information in the readings. On the basis of previous ACSM Health/Fitness Instructor certification examinations, you may receive approximately six questions from this category.

PRACTICE QUESTIONS

Instructions: Each question is followed by either four or five possible answers. Select the *best* answer to the question.

____ 1. What is obesity?

      a. a surplus of adipose tissue, containing fat stored in triglyceride form, resulting from excessive energy intake relative to energy expenditure

      b. waist girth of >100 cm

c. a BMI of ≥30 kg/m^2

d. *a* and *b*

e. *a, b,* and *c*

_____ 2. What is overweight?

a. body mass in excess of some normalized standard

b. BMI of 25.0 to 29.9 kg/m^2

c. an overfat condition

d. *a* and *b*

e. *a, b,* and *c*

_____ 3. What is lean body mass?

a. fat-free mass, including essential fat

b. the mass of the human body minus all extractable (body mass − fat mass) fat

c. body weight minus all body fat, including essential body fat

d. *a* and *b*

e. *a, b,* and *c*

_____ 4. What is the term for a serious condition, found most often among teenage girls, in which there is a loss of appetite and a possible progression to various degrees of emaciation?

a. bulimia

b. anorexia nervosa

c. negative caloric balance

d. android-type obesity

_____ 5. If one observed in a female athlete weight loss or gain, excessive concern about weight, a visit to the bathroom after meals, depression, and/or severe criticism of her own body, which of the following conditions might be expected?

a. anorexia nervosa

b. anorexia athletica

c. bulimia nervosa

d. athletica bulimia

_____ 6. In assessing obesity as a possible health risk, more than percentage of body fat should be considered. Which of the following term(s) is (are) related to a high risk for cardiovascular disease and diabetes?

    a. waist girth

    b. android-type obesity

    c. gynoid-type obesity

    d. *a* and *b*

    e. *a*, *b*, and *c*

_____ 7. Which of the following conditions may develop as a result of too much body fat?

    a. impaired cardiac function from increased mechanical work

    b. osteoarthritis; cancer of the colon

    c. hypertension and stroke

    d. *a* and *b*

    e. *a*, *b*, and *c*

_____ 8. The most effective weight loss program would include which of the following?

    a. caloric restriction and behavior modification

    b. moderate physical activity and group support

    c. aerobic exercise designed to utilize 500 kcal/day

    d. *a* and *b*

    e. *a*, *b*, and *c*

_____ 9. Caloric restriction as the sole means of weight management is *not* recommended for which of the following reasons?

    a. Fat-free mass can be lost.

    b. A decline in resting metabolic rate is observed.

    c. There is an increase in the fat storing enzyme lipoprotein lipase (LPL).

    d. *a* and *b*

    e. *a*, *b*, and *c*

_____10. Why is diet plus exercise recommended in weight loss management?

    a. Adding exercise will result in a greater fat loss.

    b. Exercise may counteract the resting metabolic decline.

    c. You can eat as much food as you like and not gain any weight.

    d. *a* and *b*

    e. *a*, *b*, and *c*

_____11. Which of the following is (are) associated with an inadequate energy intake for healthy weight management?

    a. fasting or a protein-sparing modified fast

    b. high carbohydrate/low fat

    c. low carbohydrate/high fat

    d. *a* and *b*

    e. *a*, *b*, and *c*

_____12. Which of the following could be implemented in designing a sensible weight loss plan?

    a. 500 to 1,000 kcal deficit below energy expenditure

    b. large daily deficit to lose weight rapidly

    c. undergo bariatric surgery before beginning your weight loss program

    d. *a* and *b*

    e. *a*, *b*, and *c*

_____13. Which of the following factors affect weight loss?

    a. duration of energy deficit

    b. hydration level

    c. increasing ketone body production

    d. *a* and *b*

    e. *a*, *b*, and *c*

_____14. Which of the following fat-soluble vitamins is correctly matched with function?

    a. vitamin A: facilitates blood clotting

    b. vitamin D: aids in growth and formation of bones and teeth

c. vitamin E: is important for proper reproductive function in humans

d. vitamin K: is essential in the prevention of night blindness

_____15. The following are combinations of type of vitamin, vitamin name, and conditions that result with oversupplementation. Identify the correct combination(s).

 a. water-soluble vitamin: ascorbic acid–diarrhea, kidney stones, rebound scurvy

 b. water-soluble vitamin: niacin–headaches, burning and itching skin, liver damage

 c. fat-soluble vitamin: riboflavin–cheilosis

 d. *a* and *b*

 e. *a*, *b*, and *c*

_____16. Which set correctly matches the vitamin with its functions and possible toxicity symptoms?

 a. retinol: coenzyme in CHO metabolism; loss of nerve sensation

 b. thiamin: coenzyme in energy metabolism; no observable symptoms

 c. cobalamin: maintenance of epithelial tissue; thrombosis

 d. pantothenic acid: a part of coenzyme A; diarrhea, possible kidney stones

_____17. Regarding water and exercise,

 a. exercise in hot weather increases the body's water requirement

 b. excessive sweating and large volumes of plain water may result in hyponatremia

 c. salt tablets will decrease the need for water during exercise

 d. *a* and *b*

 e. *a*, *b*, and *c*

_____18. Which of the following is a good way to determine excessive fluid loss that occurred during exercise?

 a. Measure the insensible perspiration and sweat volume on the skin.

  b. Measure water loss in the feces.

  c. Measure weight before and after exercise.

  d. Measure urine output before exercise begins.

____19. Which of the following is a (are) good suggestion(s) for fluid replacement during prolonged exercise?

  a. Ingest 300 ml of cool flavored water before exercise.

  b. During the first hour of exercise, ingest 100 to 150 ml of a cool, diluted glucose polymer.

  c. Consume a 50 percent glucose solution after one hour of exercise.

  d. *a* and *b*

  e. *a*, *b*, and *c*

____20. The Food Guide Pyramid

  a. provides foods and kcals required for optimal health

  b. provides broad recommendations for healthful nutrients

  c. has replaced the RDA

  d. is based on intensity and type of exercise

____21. Regarding calcium and health in women, which of the following is true?

  a. Osteoporosis has reached epidemic proportions in older women.

  b. Adequate calcium in the diet and exercise and resistance training can retard bone loss.

  c. Adolescents and young adults require 1,500 mg of calcium daily in the diet.

  d. *a* and *b*

  e. *a*, *b*, and *c*

____22. The following are statements characterizing the USDA Food Guide Pyramid. Which is true?

  a. Four food groups make up the Food Guide Pyramid.

  b. The majority of calories in the diet should come from the bread, cereal, rice, and pasta group; the vegetable group; and the fruit group.

    c. Because dry beans are listed in the meat category, one should consume fewer beans in the diet.

    d. Fats and oils should be consumed only if one is lactose intolerant.

_____23. Women are considered a population at risk for inadequate iron intake. Why is this true?

    a. Iron is lost during the menstrual cycle.

    b. Women do not drink enough milk.

    c. There is destruction of red blood cells via exercise.

    d. We no longer cook in iron pans and skillets.

_____24. Which of the following is (are) recommended to prevent bone loss in females?

    a. Women at high risk for osteoporosis should consume foods rich in Ca^{++}.

    b. Ca^{++} intake should be appropriate throughout life so that bone mass is optimal prior to adulthood.

    c. Women should participate in noncontact sports.

    d. *a* and *b*

    e. *a*, *b*, and *c*

_____25. Which of the following are risk factors for osteoporosis?

    a. cigarette smoking

    b. early menopause

    c. high animal protein intake

    d. *a* and *b*

    e. *a*, *b*, and *c*

_____26. Which of the following are true of dietary iron insufficiency?

    a. About 40 percent of American women of childbearing age have iron insufficiency.

    b. Dietary iron insufficiency can lead to iron deficiency anemia.

    c. Women on vegetarian diets are at greater risk because of the low bioavailability of nonheme iron.

    d. *a* and *b*

    e. *a*, *b*, and *c*

____27. Semistarvation, a part of many fad diets to promote weight loss, is not recommended because

    a. there is a loss of fat free mass

    b. one can develop malnutrition

    c. resting metabolism becomes depressed

    d. *a* and *b*

    e. *a*, *b*, and *c*

____28. Which of the following weight loss methods meet the guidelines for weight loss programs?

    a. saunas and vibrating belts

    b. programs like Weight Watchers®

    c. body wraps and sweat suits

    d. *a* and *b*

    e. *a*, *b*, and *c*

____29. Evaluation of weight loss methods has been developed and should include which of the following questions?

    a. Does the program meet my needs and are there resources to meet these needs?

    b. Is the program safe?

    c. Will the program provide long-term results and decrease obesity-related comorbities?

    d. *a* and *b*

    e. *a*, *b*, and *c*

____30. One pound of fat is equivalent to how many kilocalories?

    a. 3,086

    b. 3,500

    c. 4,086

    d. 4,500

____31. Which of the following Atwater General Factors are correct in the estimation of the energy content of foods?

    a. four kcal/gram for dietary carbohydrate

    b. four kcal/gram for dietary protein

    c. eight kcal/gram for alcohol

d. *a* and *b*

e. *a*, *b*, and *c*

____32. The lipid content of a large order of McDonald's® french fries is 21.6 grams. This is equal to how many kcals?

   a. 37.3 kcals

   b. 183.6 kcals

   c. 194.4 kcals

   d. 199.2 kcals

____33. The Atwater Factor for alcohol is

   a. four kcal/gram

   b. six kcal/gram

   c. seven kcal/gram

   d. nine kcal/gram

____34. Genetic characteristics and body fat distribution are related to

   a. the level of epinephrine secreted during exercise

   b. regional activity of lipoprotein lipase

   c. a large number of adiopocytes

   d. *a* and *b*

   e. *a*, *b*, and *c*

____35. Which of the following are indicative of regional body fat distribution and health risks?

   a. females: waist to hip ratio of >0.80 and gynoid fat patterning

   b. males: waist to hip ratio of >0.95 and android fat patterning

   c. females: waist girth measurement of >76.2 cm

   d. *a* and *b*

   e. *a*, *b*, and *c*

____36. The *female athlete triad* or the *female triad* is composed of which of the following factor(s)?

   a. amenorrhea

   b. disordered eating

c. osteoporosis

d. *a* and *b*

e. *a, b,* and *c*

_____37. Cessation of the menstrual cycle in the *female triad*

a. removes the protective element of estrogen on bone

b. decreases fertility

c. reduces urinary calcium excretion

d. leads to increases in percentage of body fat

_____38. Current information suggests that body fat distribution patterns may be associated with certain health risks. Which of the following is (are) true?

a. Those with most of their body fat in the upper body are at risk for CAD.

b. Android-type obesity poses greater health risks than gynoid-type obesity.

c. Clusters of symptoms that lead to an altered metabolic profile are associated in those who carry their fat in the trunk and abdomen.

d. *a* and *b*

e. *a, b,* and *c*

_____39. Guidelines for caloric intake for an individual desiring to lose weight would include which of the following?

a. Reduce daily intake by 500 kcals.

b. Reduce daily intake by 250 kcals and increase energy expenditure by 250 kcals.

c. Complete one day a week of complete fasting to cleanse the system of impurities.

d. *a* and *b*

e. *a, b,* and *c*

_____40. A weight loss of one pound per week is acceptable. This requires

a. reducing dietary intake by approximately 750 to 1,000 kcal

    b. reducing daily dietary intake by approximately 450 to 700 kcal and increasing energy expenditure via exercise by 300 kcal

    c. maintaining a caloric deficit of 3,500 kcals per week (500 kcals/day)

    d. obtaining a vertical band gastroplasty to "jump-start" the weight loss and proceeding with an exercise program

____41. Which of the following suggestions could be part of a program for gaining weight?

    a. Participate in a weight-training program.

    b. Increase caloric intake by a modest amount.

    c. Increase dietary protein by 14 grams/day via food.

    d. *a* and *b*

    e. *a, b,* and *c*

____42. Of the following ergogenic aids, which could actually enhance performance?

    a. bee pollen: improves metabolism and endurance performance

    b. amino acid tablets: improve gains in muscle mass

    c. ginseng: enhances energy

    d. carbohydrate loading: aids in muscle glycogen sparing

____43. Which of the following nutritional ergogenic aids is claimed to be effective for exercise tasks relying on the ATP–PC system and anaerobic glycolysis (e.g., exercise lasting one to four minutes)?

    a. carbohydrate loading

    b. bicarbonate loading

    c. glucose polymer fluid replacement drinks

    d. Gatorade®

____44. Caffeine ingestion

    a. exerts an ergogenic effect by increasing endurance capacity

    b. spares glycogen usage

      c. increases muscle cell uptake of amino acids

      d. *a* and *b*

      e. *a*, *b*, and *c*

____45. Creatine supplementation

      a. increases intramuscular Creatine and PCr

      b. enhances short-term anaerobic capacity

      c. induces heart arrhythmias in susceptible individuals

      d. *a* and *b*

      e. *a*, *b*, and *c*

____46. Nutritional factors related to the female athlete triad syndrome include which of the following viewpoints?

      a. Females who exercise heavily do not eat enough to match their caloric expenditures.

      b. Females who exercise heavily are usually anorexic.

      c. Females who exercise heavily are usually bulimic.

      d. Low fat consumption in the diet of females who exercise heavily will result in amenorrhea.

SUGGESTED READINGS

To help you demonstrate familiarity with the National Institute of Health Consensus Statement on health risks of obesity, the Nutrition for Physical Fitness Position Paper of the American Dietetic Association, Surgeon General, the National Cholesterol Education Program, and the ACSM Position Stand on proper and improper weight loss programs, we recommend the following references.

ACSM. (2003). *Official papers and opinion statements of ACSM* (16th ed.). Indianapolis: ACSM National Center. Retrieved October 7, 2003 from ACSM's Web site: http://acsm.org/publications/positionStands.htm

ADA & ACSM. (2000). Nutrition and athletic performance: Position of the American Dietetic Association, Dietitians of Canada, and the American College of Sports Medicine. *Journal of the American Dietetic Association, 100,* 1543-1556.

NIH. (1985). *Health implications of obesity*. NIH consensus statement online 1985 Feb 11-13. Retrieved June 11, 2003 from http://consensus.hih.gov/cons/049/049_statement.htm

NECP. (1993). Expert panel on detection, evaluation, and treatment of high blood cholesterol in adults. Summary of the second report of the National Cholesterol Education Program (NCEP) expert panel on detection, evaluation, and treatment of high blood cholesterol in adults (Adult Treatment Panel II). *Journal of the American Medical Association, 269,* 3015-3023.

Office of the Surgeon General. (2003). *The surgeon general's call to action prevent and decrease overweight and obesity.* Washington, DC: Superintendent of Documents, U.S. Government Printing Office. Retrieved October 7, 2003 from http://www.surgeongeneral.gov/topics/obesity/

REFERENCES FOR FURTHER STUDY

1. ACSM. (2001). *ACSM's resource manual for guidelines for exercise testing and prescription* (4th ed.). Philadelphia: Lippincott Williams & Wilkins.

2. ACSM. (2000). *ACSM's guidelines for exercise testing and prescription* (6th ed.). Philadelphia: Lippincott Williams & Wilkins.

3. McArdle, W.D., Katch, F.I., & Katch, V.I. (2001). *Exercise physiology: Energy, nutrition, and human performance* (5th ed.). Baltimore: Williams & Wilkins.

ANSWERS

Question number	Answer	KSA number	Reference	Page number
1	e	1.9.0	2	24
			1	584
2	e	1.9.0	3	753, 821, 833
3	d	1.9.0	3	762
4	b	1.9.0	3	846
5	c	1.9.0	3	846
6	e	1.9.0	3	834
			1	584
7	e	1.9.1	3	832

Question number	Answer	KSA number	Reference	Page number
8	d	1.9.2	3	841
9	d	1.9.2	3	843, 844, 852
10	d	1.9.2	1	586
			3	852
11	a	1.9.3	3	849
12	a	1.9.3	3	840
13	d	1.9.3	3	848
14	b	1.9.4	3	49, 52
15	d	1.9.4	3	49, 52
16	b	1.9.4	3	49, 58
17	d	1.9.5	3	76
18	c	1.9.5	3	76
19	d	1.9.5	1	508
20	b	1.9.6	3	86
21	e	1.9.7	3	60
22	b	1.9.6	3	85
23	a	1.9.6	3	67
24	d	1.9.7	3	61
25	e	1.9.7	3	61
26	e	1.9.7	3	67
27	e	1.9.8	3	845
28	b	1.9.8	2	481
29	e	1.9.8	1	481
30	b	1.9.10	3	851

Question number	Answer	KSA number	Reference	Page number
31	d	1.9.9	3	110
32	c	1.9.9	3	112
33	c	1.9.9	3	110
34	b	2.9.0.1	3	834
35	e	2.9.0.1	3	834
36	e	2.9.0.4	3	65
37	a	2.9.0.4	3	65
38	e	2.9.0.1	3	833
39	d	2.9.0.2	1	478
40	c	2.9.0.2	1	478
41	d	2.9.0.2	3	857
42	d	2.9.0.3	3	550, 561, 578
43	b	2.9.0.3	3	568
44	d	2.9.0.3	3	564
45	d	2.9.0.3	3	583
46	a	2.9.0.4	3	63

CHAPTER

13

Program Administration and Management

This chapter contains practice questions to test your knowledge of the ACSM certification KSAs in the category Program Administration and Management. Since this area tends to be a weakness in most applicants, you should consider setting up an appointment with an administrator to discuss these KSAs further. Fewer questions have been given to you in this section for two reasons. First, this way you will have more time to meet with an administrator. Second, questions from this section often relate to topics from other KSA categories, so a broad knowledge of information from all 10 KSA categories is as important as practice questions specifically dealing with program administration and management. It is recommended that you read section 13, *Program Management*, in *ACSM's Resource Manual for Guidelines for Exercise Testing and Prescription* (2001). On the basis of previous ACSM Health/Fitness Instructor certification examinations, you may receive approximately six questions from this category.

PRACTICE QUESTIONS

Instructions: Each question is followed by either four or five possible answers. Select the *best* answer to the question.

___ 1. Which of the following is (are) possible assignment(s) for the Health/Fitness Instructor?

    a. supervisor of programs

    b. exercise leader and programmer

    c. health counselor to the clientele

    d. supervisor of preventive programs

    e. *a*, *b*, and *c*

____ 2. Which of the following is a (are) responsibility(ies) of the Health/Fitness Instructor?

    a. reporting directly to the health/fitness facility supervisor

    b. developing exercise prescriptions and teaching classes

    c. conducting staff evaluations

    d. *a* and *b*

    e. *a*, *b*, and *c*

____ 3. As part of a Health/Fitness Instructor's responsibilities, he or she must be able to administer fitness-related programs within established budgetary guidelines. Which of the following would be profitable for a facility?

    a. providing programming not covered by dues

    b. working toward low attrition rates and high revenue-generating participants

    c. declining insurance on the facility or staff due to the tremendous drain on budget and profit

    d. *a* and *b*

    e. *a*, *b*, and *c*

____ 4. Which of the following is an (are) appropriate question(s) for formulating a marketing plan for a health/fitness facility?

    a. Examine the market environment to determine interest and needs in a facility.

    b. Identify groups and specific needs within each group.

    c. Determine profit margin.

    d. *a* and *b*

    e. *a*, *b*, and *c*

____ 5. Which of the following is a (are) good example(s) of advertising strategies?

    a. use of as many forms of media as possible

    b. repetition of the marketing message

c. free memberships

d. *a* and *b*

e. *a*, *b*, and *c*

_____ 6. A medium-sized health/fitness facility wishes to implement a new smoking-cessation program for its local community. In what promotional activities might this facility engage to maximize response and be cost-effective at the same time?

    a. Place an advertisement with a lot of white space in the newspaper to draw the attention of the reader.

    b. Depend on word of mouth from past programs.

    c. Provide for a public service announcement on one or more local radio stations to announce the new program and free lecture.

    d. *a* and *b*

    e. *a*, *b*, and *c*

_____ 7. A successful marketing approach in a health/fitness facility includes which of the following procedures?

    a. Include drop-in signups and flyers to organized groups.

    b. Determine the needs of the customer and then develop a variety of services, activities, and programs to meet those needs.

    c. Present a sales pitch to the prospective client suggesting that if the client does not participate in this program, his/her health could decline and illness and poor quality of life will eventually follow.

    d. *a* and *b*

    e. *a*, *b*, and *c*

_____ 8. Which of the following is (are) recommended for increasing sales and decreasing attrition in a health/fitness facility?

    a. Instill within the staff that customer satisfaction is every staff member's responsibility.

    b. Make sure that all promotional and sales activities are planned to occur at an appropriate time.

    c. Make the sale by any means possible.

    d. *a* and *b*

    e. *a*, *b* and *c*

_____ 9. What documentation is required to determine accountability in the event fitness facility clients have an accident or show other signs or symptoms of illness during an exercise session?

    a. job training and experience

    b. fitness test results listing important symptoms, estimation of effort, and activity demand

    c. record of equipment usage

    d. results from complete blood screening

_____10. If a client showed signs or symptoms requiring a physician's care, a variety of potential liability problems might arise. To avoid these potential problems, which of the following should be included in a facility's documentation?

    a. documentation demonstrating that critical responses to exercise were recorded

    b. documentation showing staff members who participated in emergency procedures

    c. information indicating that exercise sessions require a preexercise screening

    d. *a* and *b*

    e. *a*, *b*, and *c*

_____11. What element(s) should be included in health screening and fitness assessment forms?

    a. specific goals and objectives

    b. health appraisal questions

    c. assurance that the client carries medical insurance

    d. *a* and *b*

    e. *a*, *b*, and *c*

_____12. Which of the following would be helpful in determining participant adherence and retention in a new program?

    a. the amount of money generated as a result of the new program

    b. a survey of the current participants

    c. offering free lectures on health-related topics

    d. *a* and *b*

    e. *a*, *b*, and *c*

____13. Customer service is important in retaining members in a health/ fitness facility. What is an (are) appropriate service standard(s) for facilities?

    a. All staff members should provide world-class service from the moment a client walks in the door.

    b. Respond to members' needs as quickly as possible.

    c. Remain agreeable, friendly, and helpful when confronted by an angry member.

    d. *a* and *b*

    e. *a*, *b*, and *c*

____14. Which of the following statements is (are) true regarding the educational component in any health/fitness facility?

    a. Individuals can be instructed about the role of exercise in their lives.

    b. Any education program covering the physical, emotional, intellectual, spiritual, and social dimensions can be addressed.

    c. Free programs can be offered that can improve client retention and adherence.

    d. *a* and *b*

    e. *a*, *b*, and *c*

____15. Weight-management programs should be consistent on which of the following point(s)?

    a. All programs should sell food and nutritional supplements on site.

    b. All programs should hire a dietitian.

    c. All programs should be at least 12 weeks long in order to observe change.

    d. All programs should follow the ACSM position statement, *Proper and Improper Weight Loss Programs*.

    e. *a*, *b*, and *c*

____16. Which of the following statements is (are) true about a budget?

    a. It is a major component of long-range planning and accountability.

    b. Operating budgets require detailing goals for revenues and expenses.

    c. One assumes that expenses will increase continually.

    d. *a* and *b*

    e. *a*, *b*, and *c*

____17. For a Health/Fitness Instructor, a complete understanding of the management of the facility is important. To which of the following positions would he/she directly report?

    a. board of directors

    b. health fitness director

    c. program director

    d. fitness/wellness coordinators

    e. advisory committee

____18. Good leadership and management of employees requires

    a. that each employee know his/her exact role within the organization

    b. that each employee know what good performance looks like

    c. that each employee be allowed to do his/her job

    d. *a* and *b*

    e. *a*, *b*, and *c*

____19. To deliver sound health/fitness programs, one must be able to

    a. manage and offer a wide variety of programs and services

    b. develop appropriate business goals and objectives

    c. develop a systematic approach to programming

    d. *a* and *b*

    e. *a*, *b*, and *c*

____20. Appropriate program development requires

    a. "needs" assessments

    b. program planning

    c. program evaluation

    d. *a* and *b*

    e. *a*, *b*, and *c*

REFERENCES FOR FURTHER STUDY

1. ACSM. (2001). *ACSM's resource manual for guidelines for exercise testing and prescription* (4th ed.). Philadelphia: Lippincott Williams & Wilkins.
2. ACSM. (2000). *ACSM's guidelines for exercise testing and prescription* (6th ed.). Philadelphia: Lippincott Williams & Wilkins.

ANSWERS

Question number	Answer	KSA number	Reference	Page number
1	e	2.10.0.1	2	325
2	d	2.10.0.1	2	325
3	d	2.10.0.2	1	622
4	d	2.10.0.3	1	664
5	b	2.10.0.3	1	671
6	c	2.10.0.3	1	670
7	d	2.10.0.4	1	665
8	d	2.10.0.4	1	665
9	b	2.10.0.5	1	630
10	e	2.10.0.5	1	630
11	d	2.10.0.6	1	604
12	b	2.10.0.6	1	604
13	e	2.10.0.6	1	638
14	e	2.10.0.7	1	608
15	d	2.10.0.7	1	608
16	e	2.10.0.8	1	620
17	d	2.10.0.8	1	616
18	e	2.10.0.8	1	614

Question number	Answer	KSA number	Reference	Page number
19	e	2.10.0	1	601
20	e	2.10.0.8	1	603

14

Solving
Metabolic Equations

In addition to questions from each of the 10 ACSM KSA categories, one type of question in the written portion of the ACSM Health/ Fitness Instructor certification examination will require you to solve basic metabolic equations. The purpose of this chapter is to present a brief tutorial to the potential certification candidate. In this tutorial, you will learn how to solve metabolic equations systematically.

At the ACSM Health/Fitness Instructor level of certification, you will be required to calculate energy cost in both METs and kilocalories when the mode of exercise includes any of the following: treadmill walking, treadmill running, leg and arm ergometry, and bench stepping (see KSA category *Exercise Programming*, objectives 2.8.0.3; 2.8.0.5; 2.8.0.6; ACSM, 2000, p. 344). Table 14.1 summarizes the five metabolic equations that you will be required to use. While at first glance the metabolic equations may appear intimidating, with practice, not only will you feel your anxiety dissipating, but you will learn to enjoy the challenge that this important task offers. On the basis of previous ACSM Health/Fitness Instructor certification examinations, you are likely to receive approximately 10 questions that will require you to solve a metabolic equation.

A SYSTEMATIC APPROACH
FOR SOLVING METABOLIC EQUATIONS

As you can see in table 14.1, each metabolic equation has certain components consistent with the type of exercise used. For walking and treadmill and outdoor running, speed and grade are needed. For arm or leg ergometry, watts and body mass are required. Finally, for stepping exercises, step height and step frequency are needed. Your task will be to extract important information from a descriptive statement (the question), substitute these "knowns" (speed, grade, etc.) into the appropriate metabolic equation, and then, using principles of elementary algebra, solve for the "unknown." You can find additional examples of metabolic equations and practice problems in the *Health Fitness Instructor's Handbook* (Howley & Franks, 2003, pp. 46-58).

Table 14.1 Metabolic Equations for Oxygen Consumption ($\dot{V}O_2$) in Metric Units*

Walking	$\dot{V}O_2 = (0.1 \times S) + (1.8 \times S \times G) + 3.5$
Treadmill and outdoor running	$\dot{V}O_2 = (0.2 \times S) + (0.9 \times S \times G) + 3.5$
Leg ergometry	$\dot{V}O_2 = (10.8 \times W/M) + 7$
	$\dot{V}O_2 = 1.8 \times$ work rate (in kgm/min)/M + 7
Arm ergometry	$\dot{V}O_2 = (18 \times W/M) + 3.5$
	$\dot{V}O_2 = 3 \times$ work rate (in kgm/min)/M + 3.5
Stepping	$\dot{V}O_2\ (0.2 \times f) + (1.33 \times 1.8 \times H \times f) + 3.5$

*$\dot{V}O_2$ = ml/kg/min; S = speed in m/min; M = body mass in kg; G = percent grade written as a fraction; W = power in watts; f = frequency of stepping per minute; H = step height in meters.

The following is a list of the mathematical steps you should follow when solving any metabolic equation. It's extremely important to resist the temptation to take shortcuts; instead, get into the habit of following each and every step in this systematic approach. This will greatly reduce your chance of committing a careless error.

1. Read the descriptive statement (question) and identify important known information that you will need to substitute into the metabolic equation.

2. On a sheet of paper, write the "knowns" on the left side and the "unknown(s)" on the right side.

3. Select the appropriate metabolic equation.

4. Examine the available information to determine whether it is in the appropriate unit of measure. For example, you may be given treadmill speed (miles per hour), whereas the appropriate metabolic equation requires you to convert speed to meters per minute.

5. Using substitution, lay out the appropriate metabolic equation and solve for the unknown component.

6. Once you have solved for the unknown component, double-check to see that the answer is in the correct unit of measure and is reasonable.

Important Facts to Memorize

Initially, potential certification candidates worry needlessly about their ability to memorize all five metabolic equations. Rest assured that memorization of the metabolic equations is not necessary. As part of your examination packet, you will receive a copy of the metabolic equations as they appear on page 303 of *ACSM's Guidelines for Exercise Testing and Prescription* (ACSM, 2000). Nevertheless, while memorization is not essential, it is to your advantage to be so familiar with the equations that you do not have to consult the handout too frequently. As we pointed out in Chapter 2, you will be under a time constraint, and constantly referring to the metabolic equations handout can quickly eat up valuable time. By solving the problems presented in this chapter, you will become increasingly familiar with the structure of each equation. However, there is some information that will not be supplied to you on the exam; you must simply commit this information to memory. This essential information is presented in table 14.2.

Table 14.2   Conversion Factors

Kilocalories	1 L O_2 = 5 kcal or kcal/min/5 = $\dot{V}O_2$ ml/kg/min
Kilocalories	1 lb adipose tissue = 3,500 kcal
Weight	1 kg = 2.2 lb
Speed	26.8 × mph = m/min; 60/min/mile = mph
$\dot{V}O_2$ ml/kg/min	$\dot{V}O_2$ L/min × 1000/body mass in kg
	$\dot{V}O_2$ L/min = $\dot{V}O_2$ ml/kg/min × body mass in kg
Power	1 watt = 6.12 kgm/min (round off to 6.0 for calculations) or W × 6 = workload (kgm/min)
METs	METs × 3.5 ml/kg/min = $\dot{V}O_2$ (ml/kg/min)
METs	$\dot{V}O_2$ ml/kg/min / 3.5 = METs

SOLVING METABOLIC EQUATIONS

In this section, we provide examples that show you how to solve each of the five types of metabolic equations for *gross* $\dot{V}O_2$. Gross $\dot{V}O_2$ is total oxygen consumption, that is, rest plus exercise. You should note that in some instances you solve for gross O_2 consumption ($\dot{V}O_2$) and energy expenditure (kilocalories), while in other instances you will be given this information and asked to calculate treadmill speed, treadmill grade, cycle ergometer resistance, or some other variable.

Sometimes you will be asked to determine *net* $\dot{V}O_2$. The net oxygen consumption is the oxygen required to perform the work minus the baseline oxygen consumption of 3.5 ml/kg/min.

In the following presentation of questions and solutions, we employ the systematic approach to solving metabolic equations. Each question is answered using the step-by-step format just explained. This method may seem repetitive, but it encourages you to attack these questions in a consistent manner. This will increase your chances of success with metabolic calculations.

Walking

Walking occurs between 50 and 100 m/min (1.9-3.7 mph). No formula exist for speeds between 3.7 mph (walking) and 5.0 mph (jogging). If an individual is walking/jogging between 3.7 and 5.0 mph, you must use caution in deciding which equation to use.

Practice Question 1

What is the oxygen consumption of walking at 3.0 mph up a 2 percent grade?

Answer: 14.79 ml O_2/kg/min

1. Read the question and identify important known information.
2. Write the knowns on the left side and the unknowns on the right side.

   Known: Unknown:

   grade = 2% or 0.02 $\dot{V}O_2$(ml/kg/min)

   speed = 3.0 mph

3. Select the appropriate metabolic equation (walking).

$$\dot{V}O_2 = (0.1 \times S) + (1.8 \times S \times G) + 3.5$$

4. Examine the available information. This problem requires you to convert miles per hour to meters per minute and to convert grade to a fraction.

Convert 3.0 mph to meters per minute.

$$26.8 \text{ m/min} \times 3.0 \text{ mph} = 80.4 \text{ m/min}$$

Convert 2% to a fraction.

$$2/100 = 0.02$$

5. Using the information from above, solve for the unknowns.

$$\dot{V}O_2 \text{ ml/kg/min} = (0.1 \times 80.4) + (1.8 \times 80.4 \times 0.02) + 3.5$$
$$\dot{V}O_2 \text{ ml/kg/min} = 8.4 + 2.89 + 3.5$$
$$\dot{V}O_2 \text{ ml/kg/min} = 14.79$$

6. Double-check your answer.

Practice Question 2

An individual has set the treadmill at a 3 percent grade and 3.0 mph. Would a person wishing to exercise at approximately 5.0 METs be able to do so using these criteria?

Answer: 16.24 ml O_2/kg/min = 4.64 METs; yes

1. Read the question and identify important known information.

2. Write the knowns on the left side and the unknowns on the right side.

Known:	Unknown:
grade = 3% or 0.03	$\dot{V}O_2$ (ml/kg/min)
speed = 3.0 mph	Can subject work at 5.0 METs?

3. Select the appropriate metabolic equation (walking).

$$\dot{V}O_2 = (0.1 \times S) + (1.8 \times S \times G) + 3.5$$

4. Examine the available information. This problem requires you to convert miles per hour to meters per minute.

Convert 3.0 mph to meters per minute.

$$26.8 \text{ m/min} \times 3.0 \text{ mph} = 80.4 \text{ m/min}$$

Convert 4% to a fraction.

$$3/100 = 0.03$$

5. Using the information from above, solve for the unknowns.

$$\dot{V}O_2 = (0.1 \times 80.4) + (1.8 \times 80.4 \times 0.03) + 3.5$$
$$\dot{V}O_2 = 8.4 + 4.34 + 3.5$$
$$\dot{V}O_2 = 16.24$$

16.24 ml O_2/kg/min / 3.5 ml O_2/kg/min = 4.64 METs

Answer: yes.

6. Double-check your answer.

Practice Question 3

A cardiac patient was told by her doctor not to exercise any harder than 5 METs. At what speed (miles per hour) should this person walk if the grade is 5 percent?

Answer: 2.75 mph

1. Read the question and identify important known information.
2. Write the knowns on the left side and the unknowns on the right side.

   Known: Unknown:

   grade = 5% or 0.05 $\dot{V}O_2$ (ml/kg/min)

   METs = 5.0   speed (mph)

3. Select the appropriate metabolic equation (walking).

   $$\dot{V}O_2 = (0.1 \times S) + (1.8 \times S \times G) + 3.5$$

4. Examine the available information. This problem requires you to convert METs to $\dot{V}O_2$.

   Convert METs to $\dot{V}O_2$.

   1 MET = 3.5 ml O_2/kg/min

   5.0 × 3.5 ml/kg/min = 17.5 ml/kg/min

5. Using the available information from above, solve for the unknowns.

   a. $\dot{V}O_2 = (0.1 \times S) + (1.8 \times S \times G) + 3.5$

   17.5 = (0.1 × 26.8 m/min × S) + (1.8 × 26.8 m/min × S × 0.05) + 3.5

   Note: To convert m/min to mph use 26.8 m/min in the above equation.

$$17.5 = (2.68S) + (2.41S) + 3.5$$
$$17.5 = 5.09S + 3.5$$
$$14.0 = 5.09S$$
$$\text{Speed} = 2.75 \text{ mph}$$

6. Double-check your answer.

Treadmill Running

Jogging or running occurs at speeds greater than 134 m/min or 5.0 mph. If the person is actually jogging at 80 m/min or 3.0 mph, this equation can be used.

Practice Question 1

What is the O_2 cost of running on a treadmill at a speed of 6.0 mph and 8 percent grade?

Answer: 47.24 ml O_2/kg/min

1. Read the question and identify important known information.
2. Write the knowns on the left side and the unknowns on the right side.

   Known: Unknown:

   grade = 8.0% or 0.08 $\dot{V}O_2$ (ml/kg/min)

   speed = 6.0 mph

3. Select the appropriate metabolic equation (running).
$$\dot{V}O_2 = (0.2 \times S) + (0.9 \times S \times G) + 3.5$$

4. Examine the available information. This problem requires you to convert miles per hour to meters per minute.

   Convert miles per hour to meters per minute.
$$26.8 \text{ m/min} \times 6.0 \text{ mph} = 160.8 \text{ m/min}$$

5. Using the information from above, solve for the unknowns.
$$\dot{V}O_2 = (0.2 \times S) + (0.9 \times S \times G) + 3.5$$
$$\dot{V}O_2 = (0.2 \times 160.8 \text{ m/min}) + (0.9 \times 160.8 \text{ m/min} \times 0.08) + 3.5$$
$$\dot{V}O_2 = (32.16) + (11.58) + 3.5$$
$$\dot{V}O_2 \text{ ml/kg/min} = 47.24$$

6. Double-check your answer.

Practice Question 2

At what percent grade should the treadmill be set when a person wishes to exercise at 6 mph and 12 METs?

Answer: 4 percent

1. Read the question and identify important information.
2. Write the knowns on the left side and unknowns on the right side.

Known:	Unknown:
speed = 6 mph	$\dot{V}O_2$ (ml/kg/min)
METs = 12.0	% grade

3. Select the appropriate metabolic equations (running).

   $$\dot{V}O_2 = (0.2 \times S) + (0.9 \times S \times G) + 3.5$$

4. Examine the available information. This problem requires you to convert METs to $\dot{V}O_2$ (ml/kg/min) and miles per hour to meters per minute.

   a. Convert METs to $\dot{V}O_2$ (ml/kg/min).

   $$1\ MET = 3.5\ ml\ O_2/kg/min$$
   $$12.0 \times 3.5\ ml\ O_2/kg/min = 42.0\ ml\ O_2/kg/min$$

   b. Convert 6 mph to meters per minute.

   $$26.8 \times 6.0\ mph = 160.8\ m/min$$

5. Using the information from above, solve for the unknowns.

   $$\dot{V}O_2 = (0.2 \times S) + (0.9 \times S \times G) + 3.5$$
   $$42.0 = (0.2 \times 160.8) + (0.9 \times 160.8 \times G) + 3.5$$
   $$42.0 = (32.16) + (144.72\ G) + 3.5$$
   $$42.0 - 3.5 - 32.16 = 144.72G$$
   $$6.34 = 144.72G$$
   $$G = 0.0356\ (\text{so round to } 4\%)$$

6. Double-check your answer.

Leg Cycle Ergometry

Cycle ergometry is a non-weight-bearing activity, so typically $\dot{V}O_2$ is reported in absolute terms (L/min). However, note that in *ACSM's Guidelines for Exercise Testing and Prescription* (2002), all equations are in terms of relative $\dot{V}O_2$ (ml/kg/min). $\dot{V}O_2$ can be estimated for work rates between 50 and 200 W (300 and 1,200 kgm/min). Determination of power equals the resistance (R) = in Newtons at which the ergometer is set, times the distance (D) the flywheel travels in a single revolution (see the following text), times the number of pedal revolutions per minute (f/min). Distance (D) for the flywheel on a Monark Exercise leg cycle ergometer is 6 m/rev; the flywheel on both the Tunturi® and BodyGuard® cycle ergometers travels at 3 m/rev. Pedal revolutions are monitored with a metronome. Pedal revolutions of 50 to 60 are appropriate for untrained cyclists. For example, if you were pedaling at 50 rev/min on a Monark cycle ergometer, the distance traveled would equal 6 m/rev × 50 rev/min or 300 m/min. If a 1-kilogram force is set on the wheel, then 1 kilogram × 300 m/min = 300 kgm/min. Since 1 watt = 6 kgm/min, power would equal 50 watts.

Practice Question 1

A 143-pound male pedals a Monark cycle ergometer at 50 rev/min against a resistance of 2.0 kilograms. What is the power output? What is the relative $\dot{V}O_2$? How long would it take this individual to expend 500 kcal?

Answer: 100 watts; 23.62 ml O_2/kg/min; 65 min.

1. Read the question and identify important known information.
2. Write the knowns on the left side and the unknowns on the right side.

Known:	Unknown:
BW = 143 pounds	Power
= 65 kilograms	Vertical/resistive component
Rev/min = 50	Time to expend 500 kcal
Force = 2 kilograms	$\dot{V}O_2$ (relative)
Flywheel circumference	
= 6 m/rev	

3. Select the appropriate metabolic equations (leg cycling).

   $$\dot{V}O_2 = (10.8 \times W/M) + 7$$

4. Examine the available information. This problem requires you to determine the distance traveled for the Monark ergometer and power.

   a. Equations: distance = rev/min × m/rev; P = (F × d)/t

    b. Solve for distance.

$$\text{distance} = 50 \text{ rev/min} \times 6 \text{ m/rev}$$
$$= 300 \text{ m/min}$$

5. Using the information from the previous question, solve for the remaining unknowns.

    a. Solve for power.

Note that distance is expressed as a rate, and T = time. So if we multiply the rate (300 m/min) times the force (2 kilograms) we will be able to calculate the power output $[P = (F \times d)/t]$.

$$\text{Power} = 2 \text{ kilograms} \times 300 \text{ m/min}$$
$$\text{Power output} = 600 \text{ kgm/min}$$

Since 1 watt = 6 kgm/min, then

$$\text{Power} = 100 \text{ watts}$$

    b. Solve for $\dot{V}O_2$

$$\dot{V}O_2 = (10.8 \times 100/65) + 7$$
$$\dot{V}O_2 = 16.62 + 7$$
$$\dot{V}O_2 = 23.62 \text{ ml/kg/min}$$

    c. Time to expend 500 kcal?

Convert ml O_2/min to liters per minute.

$$23.62 \text{ ml/kg/min} = ?L$$
$$23.62 \times 65 = 1535.30 \text{ ml} = 1.54 \text{ L}$$
$$1.54 \text{ L } O_2\text{/min} \times 5 \text{ kcal/L} = 7.7 \text{ kcal/min}$$
$$500 \text{ kcal}/7.7 \text{ kcal/min} = 65 \text{ min (rounded)}$$

Therefore, it would take 65 minutes to expend 500 kcal.

6. Double-check your answer.

Alternative Equation

In *ACSM's Guidelines for Exercise Testing and Prescription* (2000, p.304) book, there is a second equation you may use for leg cycling; notice that the answer for $\dot{V}O_2$ is the same.

$$\dot{V}O_2 = 1.8 \times \text{work rate (in kgm/min)/M} + 7$$

Determine power output as you did previously.

$$\dot{V}O_2 = 1.8 \, (600 \text{ kgm/min})/65 + 7$$
$$\dot{V}O_2 = 1.8 \, (9.2) + 7$$
$$\dot{V}O_2 = 23.62 \text{ ml/kg/min}$$

Arm Cycle Ergometry

Oxygen consumption can be estimated for arm cycle ergometry for work rates between 25 and 125 watts (150 and 750 kgm/min).

Practice Question 1

A 50-kilogram female exercises on an arm cycle ergometer at 50 rev/min against a force of 25 watts. What is the absolute $\dot{V}O_2$ (ml O_2/min)?

Answer: 625 ml O_2/min.

1. Read the question and identify important known information.
2. Write the knowns on the left side and the unknowns on the right side.

Known:	Unknown:
BW = 50 kilograms	$\dot{V}O_2$ (absolute)
rev/min = 50	
power = 25 watts	

3. Select the appropriate metabolic equation (arm cycling).

   $$\dot{V}O_2 = (18 \times W/M) + 3.5$$

4. Remember, the equations are designed to give you $\dot{V}O_2$ in relative terms (ml/kg/min). The problem asks for an "absolute" value for $\dot{V}O_2$.

5. Using the information from the previous question, solve for the remaining unknowns.

   $$\dot{V}O_2 = (18 \times 25/50) + 3.5$$
   $$\dot{V}O_2 = (18 \times 0.5) + 3.5$$
   $$\dot{V}O_2 = 9 + 3.5$$
   $$\dot{V}O_2 = 12.5 \text{ (ml/kg/min)}$$

   Convert ml/kg/min to ml/min.

   $$\dot{V}O_2 = 12.5 \times 50 \text{ kg}$$
   $$\dot{V}O_2 = 625 \text{ ml } O_2/\text{min}$$

   The absolute $\dot{V}O_2$ for this arm cycle exercise is 625 ml O_2/min.

6. Double-check your answer.

Alternative Equation

In *ACSM's Guidelines for Exercise Testing and Prescription* (2000, p.304), there is a second equation you may use for arm cycling:

$$\dot{V}O_2 = 3 \times \text{work rate (in kgm/min)/M} + 3.5$$

Bench Stepping

Bench stepping is a weight-bearing activity requiring the subject to lift the body by stepping up on a box and then stepping down. The step or bench height must be converted to meters. The constant, 1.33, is used in bench-stepping exercise as it includes both the positive component of stepping up (1.0) and the negative component of stepping down (0.33). Oxygen consumption can be determined with this equation when stepping rates are between 12 and 30 steps/min and stepping heights between 0.04 and 0.4 meters.

Practice Question 1

What is the O_2 cost of bench stepping when the height of the bench is 8 inches and the stepping rate is 20?

Answer: 17.23 ml O_2/kg/min.

1. Read the question and identify important known information.
2. Write the knowns on the left side and the unknowns on the right side.

Known:	Unknown:
bench height = 8 inches	$\dot{V}O_2$
step rate = 20 steps per minute	

3. Select the appropriate metabolic equations (bench stepping).

   $$\dot{V}O_2 = (0.2 \times f) + (1.33 \times 1.8 \times H \times f) + 3.5$$

4. Examine the available information. This problem requires you to convert the bench step height in inches to meters.

   Convert bench step height in inches to meters.

   $$8 \text{ inches} \times 0.0254 \text{ meters} = 0.2032 \text{ meters}$$

5. Using the information from the previous question, solve for the remaining unknowns.

   $$\dot{V}O_2 = (0.2 \times 20) + (1.33 \times 1.8 \times 0.2032 \times 20) + 3.5$$
   $$\dot{V}O_2 = (4) + (9.73) + 3.5$$
   $$\dot{V}O_2 = 17.23$$

6. Double-check your answer.

PRACTICING CALCULATIONS

Following are 25 metabolic calculations. Work through them using the systematic approach and following the format of the examples you have used in this chapter.

1. What is the $\dot{V}O_2$ cost of exercising on a treadmill at 2.5 mph and a 6 percent grade?

2. What is the MET requirement and the caloric expenditure for an exercise session on the treadmill if you weigh 75 kilograms and want to exercise by walking at 3.7 mph up a 10 percent grade?

3. A cardiac patient cannot walk any faster than 2 mph, but she has been told that she must exercise at 8 METs. At what percent grade should the treadmill be set?

4. An elderly lady who weighs 142 pounds exercises on her treadmill at 2.5 mph. What is her caloric expenditure for a 20-minute exercise session?

5. A male who weighs 200 pounds wishes to lose weight. If he exercises on the treadmill at 3.0 mph and 10 percent grade, how long will it take to expend enough calories to equal approximately one pound?

6. If a 75-kilogram man runs at 9 mph for 30 minutes, how many kilocalories will he expend?

7. What is the O_2 cost of running at 10 mph up a 10 percent grade on a treadmill?

8. At what grade should you exercise on a treadmill if you wish to work at a 13 MET capacity? Treadmill speed is 6 mph.

9. What is the caloric cost (per minute) of the treadmill exercise in question #7? The person performing this activity weighs 55 kilograms.

10. What would be the O_2 cost of running on the level at 8 mph?

11. What is the O_2 cost of leg cycle ergometry when the workload is 400 watts and body weight is 65 kilograms?

12. What is the energy cost in METs if a person is cycling at a work rate of 300 kgm/min and weighs 50 kilograms?

13. What is the workload in watts if a person is pedaling at 60 rev/min at a resistance of 2 kilopounds on a Monark ergometer?

14. What is the absolute O_2 cost of cycling at 150 watts on a Monark cycle when the person weighs 175 pounds?

15. How long would the person in question #14 have to exercise to expend 400 kcal?

16. What is the cost in METs for a 125-pound woman who exercises at 125 watts on an arm cycle ergometer?

17. What is the O_2 cost of arm cranking at 125 watts when you weigh 80 kilograms?

18. What is the total energy expenditure for the person in question #17 after exercising for 30 minutes?

19. A man is cranking at 50 watts on the arm crank ergometer. What is his MET level? BW = 84 kg

20. A woman who weighs 95 kilograms reached 125 watts on an arm-cranking test before fatiguing. She wishes to train at 70 percent of her maximal capacity. At what work rate should she train on the arm crank ergometer?

21. What is the O_2 cost of bench stepping at a rate of 20 steps per minute when the bench is eight inches high?

22. For a 60-kilogram woman exercising on a 30-centimeter bench at a rate of 40 steps per minute, what would be the relative O_2 cost and energy expenditure in METs?

23. What is the total energy expenditure for the woman in question #22 after she has exercised for five minutes?

24. You have a client who needs preliminary testing. Your facility uses bench stepping to assess initial fitness level (bench = 6 inches; protocol uses 15 steps per minute). If your client had been told by his doctor to exercise, but *not* above 6 METs initially, could you test your client with your current protocol?

25. An individual wants to start a stair-stepping exercise routine at home. The steps are seven inches high. What stepping rate should he use if he wishes to exercise at 6 METs?

REFERENCES FOR FURTHER STUDY

1. ACSM. (2000). *ACSM's guidelines for exercise testing and prescription* (6th ed.). Philadelphia: Lippincott Williams & Wilkins.

2. Howley, E.T., & Franks, B.D. (2003). *Health fitness instructor's handbook* (4th ed.). Champaign, IL: Human Kinetics.

3. Kaminsky, L.A. (2001). *ACSM's metabolic calculations tutorial CD-ROM*. (Version 1.0a). Philadelphia: Lippincott Williams & Wilkins.

ANSWERS

1	17.44 ml O_2/kg/min
2	8.93 METs; 11.75 kcal/min
3	19.8% or 20%
4	65.84 kcal in 20 minutes
5	Approximately five hours
6	582 kcal in 30 minutes
7	81.22 ml O_2/kg/min
8	.068% or 7%
9	22.34 kcal/min
10	46.38 mlO_2/kg/min
11	73.96 ml/kg/min
12	4.68 METs
13	120 watts
14	2176 ml O_2/min
15	36.76 minutes
16	12.3 METs
17	31.63 ml/kg/min or 2,530 ml O_2/min
18	379.5 kcal for 30 minutes
19	4.06 METs
20	87.5 watts or 525 kgm/min
21	17.07 ml O_2/kg/min
22	40.23 ml O_2/kg/min; 11.5 METs
23	60.4 kcal for five minutes

24	Yes, protocol requires 3.4 METs
25	28 steps per minute

15

Analyzing
Case Studies

Most of the study questions you have seen so far have been presented in a straightforward manner. You have simply been asked to respond to specific questions in a multiple-choice format. However, when working in a real-world setting, the exercise professional must learn to make decisions based on an array of information. This information is generally obtained through such means as medical history, blood profile analyses, physical examination, and exercise test results. Collectively, this information is referred to as a case study. Your job as an exercise professional is to consider all available information in making your exercise recommendations. Listed are some of the questions the exercise professional may ask when analyzing the information in a client's file.

- What is the client's risk stratification?
- Does the client exhibit major signs or symptoms suggestive of cardiopulmonary or metabolic disease?
- Is the client taking any medications? If so, what effect, if any, do the medications have on the exercise response?
- Are blood chemistry profiles in line with suggested recommendations?
- Did the client exhibit a normal HR and BP response to exercise?
- What is the client's true functional capacity? How does this information affect the establishment of a target HR range?
- Should the client be placed in a supervised or an unsupervised program?

- Does the client exhibit any orthopedic or other exercise-related limitations?
- What would be the most appropriate mode of exercise for this client?

In this chapter, you will have the opportunity to review four case studies. We suggest that after studying each case file you attempt to formulate your own series of important questions before answering the questions we have supplied. If you would like additional practice in analyzing case studies, consult *Exercise Prescription: A Case Study Approach to the ACSM Guidelines* (Swain and Leutholtz, 2002).

CASE STUDY 1

Paul is a male who is 36 years of age, weighs 88 kilograms, is 178 centimeters tall, and has 28 percent body fat. Blood chemistry values indicated that TC = 270 mg/dl and HDL-C = 38 mg/dl. Paul's mother died of a heart attack at the age of 63, and his father had a heart attack at the age of 68. Paul is sedentary and has engaged in no endurance-training program since college. Table 15.1 shows the results of his maximal GXT, conducted by his physician.

Table 15.1   Test: Balke, 3 mi × hr^{-1}, 2.5% per 2 min

Grade %	METs	SBP	DBP	HR	ECG	Symptoms
	Rest	126	88	70	—	—
2.5	4.3	142	86	142	—	—
5	5.4	148	88	150	—	—
7.5	6.4	162	86	160	—	—
10	7.4	174	84	168	—	—
12.5	8.5	186	84	176	—	—
15	9.5	194	84	190	—	Calf tight
17.5	10.5	198	84	198	—	Fatigue

Reprinted, by permission, from E.T. Howley and B.D. Franks, 2003, *Health fitness instructor's handbook,* 2nd ed. (Champaign, IL: Human Kinetics), 187.

___ 1. What is the approximate range of Paul's target HR, in beats per minute, based on 60 to 80 percent $\dot{V}O_2max$?

  a. 122 to 135

  b. 135 to 152

  c. 139 to 168

  d. 158 to 175

___ 2. Paul's target HR range as calculated in problem #1 corresponds to what work rate range in METs?

  a. 1.5 to 3.5

  b. 2.5 to 5.0

  c. 6.3 to 8.4

  d. 8.6 to 9.5

___ 3. What is revealed by Paul's medical history and blood profile?

  a. a positive family history for CAD

  b. a significantly elevated HDL-C value

  c. an HDL-C level that is below the minimal recommendation

  d. a TC : HDL-C ratio of 7.1

___ 4. What is revealed by Paul's GXT results?

  a. a true functional capacity of 9.5 METs

  b. a true functional capacity of 10.5 METs

  c. an elevated resting BP

  d. an abnormal DBP response during exercise

CASE STUDY 2

Mary is a 38-year-old female who is 170 centimeters tall, weighs 61.4 kilograms, and has 39 percent body fat. Blood chemistry values indicate a TC of 188 mg/dl and an HDL-C of 59 mg/dl. Her resting BP is 124/80. Family history indicates that her father suffered a nonfatal heart attack at the age of 67. Mary has smoked one pack of cigarettes a day for the past 13 years. The results of her submaximal cycle ergometer test are shown in table 15.2.

Table 15.2 Test: Y Way of Fitness

Work rate (kgm · min⁻¹)	HR (Min 2)	HR (Min 3)
150	118	120
300	134	136

Note: Pedal rate = 50 rpm; predicted HR max = 182 beats · min⁻¹; seat height = 6; 85% HR max = 155 beats · min⁻¹.

Reprinted, by permission, from E.T. Howley and B.D. Franks, 2003, *Health fitness instructor's handbook*, 2nd ed. (Champaign, IL: Human Kinetics), 187.

___ 5. What does Mary's blood lipid profile indicate?

    a. a TC : HDL-C ratio of approximately 4.1

    b. a high HDL-C value

    c. an elevated TC value

    d. *b* and *c*

    e. none of these

___ 6. Mary wishes to reduce her percentage of body fat to 22. What would be her corresponding target body weight?

    a. 50 kilograms

    b. 55 kilograms

    c. 121 pounds

    d. 130 pounds

___ 7. What is revealed by Mary's medical history?

    a. a positive health history for the development of CAD

    b. a need to participate in a smoking-cessation program

    c. a need to elevate her HDL-C

    d. a need to lower TC

CASE STUDY 3

Chris is a female, 49 years of age, who is 164 centimeters tall, weighs 93 kilograms, and has 40 percent body fat. Her serum TC is 190 mg/dl, serum triglycerides are 100 mg/dl, blood glucose is 92 mg/dl, and resting BP is 130/84. In college she was active in swimming and tennis, but since then she has had a relatively sedentary lifestyle. Her goal is to lose weight and become active again. Table 15.3 shows the results of a submaximal GXT taken to 85 percent of predicted maximal HR.

Table 15.3   Test: Balke, 3 mi × hr^{-1}, 2.5% per 2 min

Grade %	METs	SBP (mmHg)	DBP (mmHg)	HR	RPE
2.5	4.3	134	90	122	11
5	5.4	140	90	132	13
7.5	6.4	162	80	143	14

Note: Predicted HR max = 171 beats · min^{-1} and 85% HR max = 145 beats · min^{-1}.
Reprinted, by permission, from E.T. Howley and B.D. Franks, 1992, *Health fitness instructor's handbook,* 2nd ed. (Champaign, IL: Human Kinetics), 253.

___ 8. What is the most appropriate mode of activity for Chris, given that she wants to become more active and lose weight?

   a. a sport such as basketball, which she enjoys

   b. walking and/or swimming

   c. jogging

   d. high-impact aerobic stepping

___ 9. What is revealed by information from Chris' case file?

   a. It is likely that she has diabetes.

   b. She has an elevated serum triglyceride level.

   c. She has a TC : HDL-C ratio of 1.9.

   d. She exhibited normal HR, BP, and RPE response during exercise.

CASE STUDY 4

A 28-year-old female police officer (5 feet 5 inches, 140 pounds, 28 percent body fat) has enrolled in the adult fitness program. Her job demands a fairly high level of physical fitness, a level she was able to achieve six years ago when she passed the physical fitness test battery used by the police department.

   Before becoming a police officer, the client jogged 20 minutes, usually three times a week. Since starting this job, she has had little or no time for exercise and has gained 15 pounds. She works eight hours a day, is divorced, and takes care of two children, ages 7 and 9.

At least three times a week, she and the children dine out, usually at fast-food restaurants like Kentucky Fried Chicken, Burger King, or Taco Bell. She reports that her job, along with the sole responsibility for raising her children, is quite stressful. Occasionally she experiences headaches and a tightness in the back of her neck. Usually in the evening she has a glass of wine to relax.

Her medical history reveals that she smoked one pack of cigarettes a day for four years while she was in college. She quit smoking three years ago. For the past two years, she has tried some quick weight-loss diets, with little success. She was hospitalized twice to give birth to her children. She reports that her father died of heart disease when he was 52 and that her older brother has high BP.

Recently, the client had her blood chemistry analyzed because she was feeling light-headed and dizzy after eating. In an attempt to lose weight, she eats only one large meal a day, at dinnertime. Results of the blood analysis were TC = 220 mg/dl; triglycerides = 98 mg/dl; glucose = 82 mg/dl; HDL = 37 mg/dl; and TC : HDL ratio = 5.9.

The exercise evaluation yielded the data in the following list and in table 15.4:

Mode/Protocol: Treadmill/Modified Bruce

Resting data: Heart rate = 75 bpm

BP = 140/82 mmHg

Table 15.4 Data Accumulated During Case Study 4

Stage	Workload (METs)	Duration (min)	HR (beats/min)	BP (mmHg)	RPE
1	2.3	3	126	145/78	8
2	3.5	3	142	160/78	11
3	4.6	3	165	172/80	14
4	7.0	3	190	189/82	18

Endpoint: Stage 4 (2.5 mph, 12% grade). Terminated because of fatigue. No significant ST-segment depression or arrhythmias.

Reprinted, by permission, from V.H. Heyward, 2002, *Advanced fitness assessment and exercise prescription,* 2nd ed. (Champaign, IL: Human Kinetics), 104.

___ 10. What is the number of major CAD risk factors present in this client's CAD risk profile?

    a. none

    b. one

    c. two

    d. three

    e. more than three

___ 11. What is this client's initial risk stratification?

    a. low risk

    b. moderate risk

    c. high risk

    d. grave risk

___ 12. Which of the following is *not* an independent positive CAD risk factor?

    a. family history

    b. hypercholesterolemia

    c. high HDL

    d. obesity

___ 13. What is revealed by this client's GXT results?

    a. a functional aerobic capacity of approximately 24.5 ml × kg/min

    b. an abnormal DBP response to exercise

    c. a abnormal SBP response between stage 3 and stage 4 of the GXT

    d. none of these

___ 14. If this client were to participate in an outdoor walking program, on a level track, at a training intensity of 60 percent of VO_2 max, what would be her walking speed?

    a. 11 minutes, 22 seconds/mile

    b. 12 minutes, 44 seconds/mile

    c. 14 minutes, 16 seconds/mile

    d. 15 minutes, 32 seconds/mile

REFERENCES FOR FURTHER STUDY

1. Heyward, V.H. (1991). *Advanced fitness assessment and exercise prescription* (2nd ed.). Champaign, IL: Human Kinetics.
2. Howley, E.T., & Franks, B.D. (1992). *Health fitness instructor's handbook* (2nd ed.). Champaign, IL: Human Kinetics.
3. Howley, E.T., & Franks, B.D. (1997). *Health fitness instructor's handbook* (3rd ed.). Champaign, IL: Human Kinetics.
4. Swain, D.P., & Leutholtz, B.C. (2002). *Exercise prescription: A case study approach to the ACSM guidelines.* Champaign, IL: Human Kinetics.

ANSWERS

Question number	Answer	Reference	Page number
1	d	3	478
2	c	3	478
3	d	3	42
4	b	3	288
5	e	3	478
6	b	3	478
7	b	3	478
8	b	2	253
9	d	2	253
10	e	1	279
11	b	1	279
12	c	1	279
13	a	1	279-280
14	c	1	281

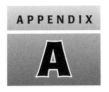
The Practice Examination

This appendix consists of a practice written examination that contains 115 questions. We encourage you to take this practice examination during one three-hour sitting. This will allow you to become familiar with, and thus prepare you for, the feelings you are likely to experience during the actual certification examination.

In appendix B, on pages 233-238, you will find an answer sheet for the practice exam. Enter the appropriate answer for each question in the first blank next to the question number. Use the second column of blank lines for correcting your practice examination. Fill in the correct answer for each question you answered incorrectly. This will make it easy for you to determine the areas in which you need to improve.

Two sets of answers are furnished at the end of the practice examination. The first set is a sequential answer list (#1- #115), while the second provides answers broken down by KSA category. This second answer set will allow you to better identify categories of strength and weakness. You should strive to obtain at least 80 percent in each of the KSA categories before attempting ACSM certification (even though ACSM standards for passing are lower).

ACSM HEALTH/FITNESS INSTRUCTOR PRACTICE EXAMINATION

Instructions: Each question is followed by either four or five possible answers. Select the *best* answer to the question.

1. What is the term that describes the volume of blood pumping through the aorta each minute?

   a. stroke volume

   b. cardiac output

   c. ejection fraction

   d. end-systolic volume

2. What is the immediate source of energy for muscular work?

   a. ATP-PC system

   b. anaerobic glycolysis

   c. aerobic glycolysis

   d. oxidative phosphorylation

3. Why is children's ability to thermoregulate during heat exposure less efficient than that of adults?

   a. Children have a higher threshold for the onset of sweating, a higher skin blood flow, a higher sweat output rate from heat-activated sweat glands, and a larger surface area to body mass ratio.

   b. Children have a higher threshold for the onset of sweating, a lower skin blood flow, a lower sweat output rate from heat-activated sweat glands, and a larger surface area to body mass ratio.

   c. Children have a lower threshold for the onset of sweating, a lower skin blood flow, a higher sweat output rate from heat-activated sweat glands, and a smaller surface area to body mass ratio.

   d. Children have a lower threshold for the onset of sweating, a higher skin blood flow, a lower sweat output rate from heat-activated sweat glands, and a smaller surface area to body mass ratio.

4. How should the exercise professional deal with a participant who overexerts him/herself during an exercise session?

   a. Recognize the potential liability that this person presents to the program and immediately drop the participant from the program.

   b. Explain to the participant the potential dangers associated with exercising above one's target HR.

   c. Suspend the participant's exercise facility privileges for one week.

d. Assign a staff member to exercise with this individual on a full-time basis to ensure that the participant will not over-exert him/herself.

e. *b* and *d*

5. What instructions should the exercise professional give to a participant who is about to perform the sit-and-reach test?

a. Bounce to reach farther on the measurement scale.

b. Remove shoes before testing.

c. Perform two trials to provide two scores that will be recorded as an average.

d. Inhale and drop the head between the arms when reaching forward.

e. *b* and *d*

6. Which of the following is a (are) negative CAD risk factor(s)?

a. hypertension

b. diabetes

c. high serum HDL-C

d. *a* and *b*

7. An elderly woman is walking on the treadmill. Suddenly, she feels light-headed and calls for your help. You notice that her speech is slurred and she is about to collapse. What do you do first?

a. Call the EMS.

b. Call the EMS, then immediately go to the door and wait for the emergency squad.

c. Immediately place the victim on the floor and check the airway and circulation.

d. *a* and *b*

e. *a*, *b*, and *c*

8. 12 METs equal a $\dot{V}O_2$ of

a. 37 ml/kg/min

b. 42 ml/kg/min

c. 45 ml/kg/min

d. 51 ml/kg/min

9. Match the food/food group with the appropriate caloric content.

a. alcohol: 9 kcal/gram

b. carbohydrate: 8 kcal/gram

c. fat: 9 kcal/gram

d. protein: 8 kcal/gram

10. What role in administration and program management does the Health/Fitness Instructor have?

a. scheduling fitness programs and staff to conduct classes

b. developing variety with respect to fitness classes

c. training new staff members

d. *a* and *b*

e. *a*, *b*, and *c*

11. Which of the following muscles adducts, medially rotates, and extends the arm?

a. latissimus dorsi

b. infraspinatus

c. pectoralis major

d. triceps brachii

12. What supplies ATP during long-term (10- to 60-minute) exercise?

a. aerobic metabolism of CHO

b. aerobic metabolism of fat

c. aerobic metabolism of fat and CHO

d. aerobic metabolism of protein

13. Which of the following is true with regard to HR in an elderly population?

a. It tends to decline, and maximal HR tends to decrease.

b. It tends to increase, and maximal HR increases in men but decreases in women.

c. It shows little to no change, and maximal HR tends to decrease.

d. It increases in women but decreases in men, and maximal HR tends to decrease in both men and women.

14. Which of the following is considered the most effective method for changing health behaviors?

   a. goal-setting

   b. reinforcement

   c. shaping

   d. stimulus-control

15. When taking a blood pressure, at what mmHg should the cuff be inflated above the SBP?

   a. 10

   b. 20

   c. 30

   d. 40

   e. 50

16. Exercise can change cholesterol levels. Which of the following statements is (are) true regarding the change observed in cholesterol?

   a. increase in HDL-C

   b. increase in both HDL-C and LDL-C

   c. increase in LDL-C

   d. *a* and *b*

   e. *a, b,* and *c*

17. Which of the following would be recommended for the immediate care of a client who is observed with dyspnea?

   a. rest and elevate the feet

   b. lay the person on the floor and check for circulation and an open airway

   c. use the AED to alleviate the problem and activate the EMS

   d. *a* and *b*

   e. *a, b,* and *c*

18. What is the recommended exercise intensity for individuals older than 65 years of age?

   a. 55/60 to 90 percent of HR max

   b. 55/60 to 90 percent of HRR

c. 55/60 to 90 percent of $\dot{V}O_{2\,R}$

d. 55/60 to 90 percent of HRR max

19. Eating disorders are prominent among

a. female athletes

b. male athletes

c. those with menstrual dysfunction

d. *a* and *b*

e. *a*, *b*, and *c*

20. For an exercise professional, what is the first step in working with an apparently healthy 35-year-old male who is interested in beginning a low- to moderate-intensity exercise program?

a. administering the Physical Activity Readiness Questionnaire

b. asking a client to obtain a physician's clearance before beginning a program

c. contacting the individual's cardiologist to obtain permission for GXT

d. giving the Cooper 12-minute run test

21. Which muscles flex the forearm?

a. the biceps brachii

b. the brachialis

c. the brachioradialis

d. *a* and *b*

e. *a*, *b*, and *c*

22. What term is given to the amount of blood pumped out of the heart with every beat?

a. stroke volume

b. ejection fraction

c. end-systolic volume

d. cardiac output

23. Which of the following is true regarding children and training?

a. Excessive endurance exercise could place a prepubescent child at increased risk for a decrease in height.

b. Children should *not* be permitted to perform maximum lifts (1RM) until reaching a Tanner stage 3 level of maturity.

c. Prepubescent children who regularly participate in a weight-training program generally demonstrate increased strength with moderate muscle hypertrophy.

d. ACSM guidelines recommend that young children perform resistance-training exercise no more than two days per week.

24. To enhance exercise adherence, what should the exercise professional communicate to the exercise participant?

a. the need to continue exercising even when not feeling well, since even one missed exercise session can lead to long-term noncompliance

b. the need to develop a relapse-prevention strategy prior to the start of the exercise program

c. the appropriateness of a sense of guilt after missing an exercise session

d. the need to realize that after missing an exercise session, it will be necessary to work twice as hard in the next session in order to make up for the missed session

25. What are associated with excessive amounts of abdominal fat?

a. hypertension, type 1 diabetes, hyperlipidemia, and CAD

b. hypertension, type 1 diabetes, hypolipidemia, and CAD

c. hypotension, type 2 diabetes, hypolipidemia, and CAD

d. hypertension, type 2 diabetes, hyperlipidemia, and CAD

26. Select the statement that best describes Mr. Vern's cholesterol and lipoprotein profile based on the following data: 34 years old; TC 210 mg/dl; LDL-C 130 mg/dl; HDL-C 34 mg/dl; serum triglycerides 300 mg/dl.

a. TC, LDL-C, HDL-C, and serum triglycerides are all borderline high.

b. TC, HDL-C, and serum triglycerides are all borderline high, while LDL-C is within the desired range.

c. TC and serum triglycerides are borderline high, while LDL-C and HDL-C are within a desirable range.

    d. TC, LDL-C, and serum triglycerides are all borderline high, while HDL-C is too low.

27. Musculoskeletal injuries are likely to occur with what type of training?

    a. training according to unsound principles

    b. training that involves high frequency and volume

    c. training seven days a week for three to four hours a day

    d. *a* and *b*

    e. *a*, *b*, and *c*

28. Besides the low back, what other area of muscle is associated with a lack of flexibility in chronic low back pain?

    a. anterior thigh

    b. posterior thigh

    c. tibialis anterior

    d. soleus

29. Which of the following conclusions from research studies support(s) the notion that exercise is prescribed as an important component in weight management?

    a. The cumulative effects of exercise on energy expenditure can be significant.

    b. Exercise and its effects may repress the appetite.

    c. Exercise may minimize the loss of lean body mass.

    d. *a* and *b*

    e. *a*, *b*, and *c*

30. What element(s) should be contained in health screening and fitness forms?

    a. a diagnosis of any health problems the client may have

    b. health appraisal questions

    c. an outline of the emergency procedure that will be followed

    d. *a* and *b*

    e. *a*, *b*, and *c*

31. Which of the following muscles contribute(s) to knee extension?

    a. quadriceps femoris

    b. rectus femoris, vastus lateralis, vastus medialis, vastus intermedius

    c. hamstring muscles and sartorius

    d. *a* and *b*

    e. *a*, *b*, and *c*

32. What is the end product of glycolysis that results during non-aerobic exercise?

    a. pyruvate

    b. lactate

    c. lactate dehydrogenase

    d. phosphoenolpyruvate

33. How do exercise and relaxation training compare for managing stress?

    a. Relaxation training is more effective than exercise.

    b. Exercise training is more effective than relaxation training.

    c. Exercise and relaxation training are equally effective.

    d. A combination of exercise and relaxation training is most effective.

34. Match the drug with its class of action.

    a. β-blocker: antihypertensive agent

    b. Quinidine: antiarrhythmic agent

    c. Digitoxin: diuretic agent

    d. *a* and *b*

    e. *a*, *b*, and *c*

35. A client complains of shoulder and arm pain at rest and especially during exercise. This discomfort has developed gradually over the past two years. The client believes the pain is a simple muscle strain from shoveling snow. What should you do based on your client's complaint?

a. Allow the client to continue aerobic activity (running), but discourage the use of resistance training until the pain has subsided.

b. Allow the client to continue aerobic activity (jogging) and lower-body resistance training, but discontinue upper-body resistance training until the pain has subsided.

c. Instruct the client to perform 10 extra minutes of shoulder and arm flexibility exercise before engaging in an established exercise routine.

d. Require the client to receive physician's clearance before engaging in physical activity.

36. Which of the following exercises would be beneficial to a patient with low back problems?

a. aerobic exercise

b. straight-leg sit-ups

c. leg raises

d. the plough

37. Which of the following flexibility exercises is (are) designed to stretch the gastrocnemius, hamstrings, and erector spinae?

a. modified hurdler's stretch

b. sitting toe touch

c. side bend

d. *a* and *b*

e. *b* and *c*

38. Inadequate iron intake frequently occurs in

a. young children

b. teenagers

c. young women of child-bearing age

d. *a* and *b*

e. *a*, *b*, and *c*

39. Which of the following is a recommended concept to increase sales and decrease attrition at a health/fitness facility?

a. Promise the client anything in order to complete the sale.

b. Customer satisfaction is required of all staff.

c. Point out to the client that the exercise program provided by the facility might save his/her life.

d. To decrease overcrowding, do not allow drop-ins at the facility.

40. Which muscles are located in the posterior thigh?

a. the hamstring muscles

b. the biceps femoris, semimembranosus, and semitendinosus

c. the rectus femoris, vastus lateralis, and vastus medialis

d. *a* and *b*

e. *a*, *b*, and *c*

41. Which one of the following activities comes closest to an energy expenditure of 10 METs?

a. archery

b. badminton

c. cricket

d. golf with motorized golf cart

e. running a 10-minute mile

42. DOMS is most likely due to which of the following mechanisms?

a. lactate accumulation in the muscle

b. microscopic tears in the muscle fibers

c. muscle spasms

d. *a* and *b*

e. *a*, *b*, and *c*

43. The informed consent form for an exercise test should include

a. the purpose and explanation of the test

b. an explanation or list of the risks and discomforts

c. a statement regarding the patient's freedom to stop the test

d. *a* and *b*

e. *a*, *b*, and *c*

44. The atherosclerotic process is initiated when injury to the arterial wall is sustained in which tissue layer?
    a. adventitia
    b. endothelium
    c. intima
    d. lamina
    e. media

45. One of your female clients has osteoporosis and wants to begin a flexibility program. How would you help this client?
    a. Encourage her to stretch through the limits of the normal ROM.
    b. Warn her to stretch with caution.
    c. Help her to set individual goals.
    d. *a* and *b*
    e. *a*, *b*, and *c*

46. Which of the following are considered contraindications for exercising during pregnancy?
    a. pregnancy-induced hypertension
    b. preterm rupture of membrane
    c. one maximal test already completed during pregnancy
    d. *a* and *b*
    e. *a*, *b*, and *c*

47. Of the following vitamins, which water-soluble vitamin is correctly matched with its function?
    a. B_1–thiamine: a coenzyme of energy metabolism
    b. B_6–riboflavin: facilitates mechanism in energy metabolism
    c. folic acid–B complex: a coenzyme in nucleic acids and protein synthesis
    d. biotin–B complex: a coenzyme in CHO and fat metabolism

48. Which of the following are required when developing a fitness program?
    a. program planning
    b. program evaluation

c. flyers and sales on services to encourage the community to join

d. *a* and *b*

e. *a*, *b*, and *c*

49. Which of the following is true regarding wearing light (<0.45 kilograms) ankle weights during walking or running exercise?

   a. It will not alter lower-extremity ROM.

   b. It appreciably alters lower-extremity ROM.

   c. It increases the risk of injury to the ankle joint.

   d. It is not contraindicated for individuals with orthopedic problems.

50. What is the primary energy source for performing short-term, high-intensity activity?

   a. anaerobic sources

   b. the ATP-PC system when the activity is a 400-meter dash (lasting 45 seconds)

   c. anaerobic glycolysis when the activity is a football play

   d. *a* and *b*

   e. *a*, *b*, and *c*

51. What should the exercise professional use to palpate the radial pulse?

   a. the thumb

   b. the thumb and first finger

   c. the first two fingers

   d. a stethoscope

52. Which of the following may cause coronary artery injury?

   a. viral infections

   b. hypercholesterolemia

   c. beta blockers

   d. *a* and *b*

   e. *a*, *b*, and *c*

53. Regarding skeletal muscle and strength, which of the following statements is (are) true?
    a. The proportion of fast- and slow-twitch fibers an individual has is determined at birth.
    b. Muscle function decreases 25 percent by the age of 65 years.
    c. There is little evidence to suggest that resistance training is of value for an elderly individual.
    d. *a* and *b*
    e. *a*, *b*, and *c*

54. What mode of prolonged exercise is most likely to produce improvement in $\dot{V}O_2$max?
    a. nonrhythmic large-muscle activity
    b. nonrhythmic small-muscle activity
    c. rhythmic large-muscle activity
    d. rhythmic small-muscle activity

55. Thirst lags behind the body's need for water. Which of the following is (are) used to prevent dehydration?
    a. drinking one cup of water every 15 minutes during exercise
    b. consuming 200 to 400 milliliters of water every 20 minutes during exercise
    c. consuming 500 milliliters of water every 30 minutes during exercise
    d. *a* and *b*
    e. *a*, *b*, and *c*

56. A Health/Fitness Instructor must be diligent in working within a set budget. Which of the following examples might be appropriate for meeting budget guidelines?
    a. Lock storage cabinets that contain supplies and other goods and limit key distribution.
    b. Provide a means to restrict unlimited use the copy machine.
    c. Pay attention to pricing on items from vendors; make note of increases; asks for price lists periodically.

d. *a* and *b*

e. *a*, *b*, and *c*

57. Movements of elevation, depression, abduction, adduction, upward rotation, and downward rotation can all be found in which joint?

   a. hip

   b. shoulder

   c. wrist

   d. ankle

58. Which statement(s) is (are) true about short-term, high-intensity exercise?

   a. ATP is supplied primarily from aerobic sources.

   b. A half-mile swim is a good example of this type of activity.

   c. In events lasting between 5 and 60 seconds, ATP is supplied primarily supplied by the ATP-PC system and anaerobic glycolysis.

   d. *a* and *b*

   e. *a*, *b*, and *c*

59. Of the five Korotkoff sounds (phases), which is considered to represent DBP in adults?

   a. 1

   b. 2

   c. 3

   d. 4

   e. 5

60. Regular physical activity performed by an older adult on most days of the week

   a. reduces the risk of developing or dying from some of the leading causes of illness and death

   b. reduces the risk of developing diabetes

   c. increases strength and thereby decreases falls

   d. *a* and *b*

   e. *a*, *b*, and *c*

61. Which of the following best describes the ACSM exercise prescription guideline for improving muscular strength and endurance?

  a. three sets of 8 to 10 exercises designed to train the major muscle groups, performed at least four days per week, using 8 to 12 repetitions per set

  b. one set of 8 to 10 exercises designed to train the major muscle groups, performed at least two days per week, using 4 to 8 repetitions per set

  c. three sets of 8 to 10 exercises designed to train the major muscle groups, performed at least three days per week, using 8 to 12 repetitions per set

  d. one set of 8 to 10 exercises designed to train the major muscle groups, performed at least two days per week, using 8 to 12 repetitions per set

62. Several hypotheses have been developed to explain the role of exercise in the prevention or treatment of low back pain. Which of the following are acceptable hypotheses?

  a. Exercise stimulates tissue hypertrophy.

  b. Exercise is a better treatment than surgery or bed rest.

  c. Exercise benefits disc nutrition.

  d. *a* and *b*

  e. *a*, *b*, and *c*

63. The important components of an individualized exercise prescription include which of the following?

  a. appropriate mode and intensity

  b. appropriate frequency and duration

  c. appropriate progression

  d. *a* and *b*

  e. *a*, *b*, and *c*

64. The amount of movement within a specific joint (ROM) is limited by which of the following?

  a. the bony structures of two articulating surfaces

  b. the length of the ligaments

  c. the length of the bone

d. *a* and *b*

e. *a*, *b*, and *c*

65. Isometric exercise may present hazards to the participant. Which of the following might be viewed as more of a risk with isometric as compared to isotonic exercise?

   a. increase in left ventricular wall pressure loading; increase in DBP

   b. increase in HR; increase in SBP

   c. increase in left ventricular wall pressure loading; increase in rate-pressure product; increase in SBP

   d. increase in left ventricular wall volume loading; increase in SBP; increase in DBP

66. For which of the following individuals would medical clearance be warranted before the administration of an exercise test?

   a. a 25-year-old male with one CAD risk factor (no signs or symptoms) who wishes to perform vigorous exercise

   b. a 25-year-old female with two CAD risk factors (no signs or symptoms) who wishes to perform vigorous exercise

   c. a 33-year-old female, diagnosed two years ago with non-insulin-dependent diabetes with no additional CAD risk factors (no signs or symptoms), who wishes to perform vigorous exercise

   d. *a* and *c*

   e. *a*, *b* and *c*

67. The potential limitation(s) to prolonged exercise in children include(s) which of the following?

   a. heat intolerance

   b. low sweat rate

   c. limited cardiovascular response to exercise

   d. *a* and *c*

   e. *a*, *b* and *c*

68. What do ACSM exercise prescription guidelines suggest for improving flexibility?

   a. stretching at least two days per week, holding each stretch for 75 to 90 seconds, and performing three to five repetitions for each dynamic stretch

   b. stretching at least two days per week, holding each stretch for 60 to 90 seconds, and performing one to two repetitions for each static stretch

   c. stretching at least three days per week, holding each stretch for 45 to 60 seconds, and performing one to two repetitions for each dynamic stretch

   d. stretching at least three days per week, holding each stretch for 10 to30 seconds, and performing three to five repetitions for each static stretch

69. Regarding bone mass density (BMD) across the life span, which of the following statements are true?

   a. Peak bone mass occurs in the second decade of life.

   b. Peak bone mass is higher in boys and men and the rate of loss is not as severe as what is observed in women.

   c. Postmenopausal women demonstrate little change in BMD with resistance exercise.

   d. *a* and *b*

   e. *a, b,* and *c*

70. The National Association for Sport and Physical Education has developed activity guidelines for children. Which of the following are considered appropriate guidelines for children?

   a. Elementary school-aged children should accumulate 30 to 60 minutes of sustained physical activity on most or all days of the week.

   b. Elementary school-aged children should accumulate 30 to 60 minutes of intermittent physical activity on most or all days of the week.

   c. Elementary school-aged children should accumulate 20 minutes of intermittent physical activity on most or all days of the week.

d. Elementary school-aged children should accumulate 20 minutes of sustained physical activity on most or all days of the week.

71. Which of the following is (are) a common foot strike pattern(s) in running?

    a. striking the ground with rear foot; subtalar joint in supination; pronation

    b. striking the ground at midfoot; slight backward motion; toe-off

    c. striking the ground on toe; falling back on heel; rolling foot lateral to medial

    d. *a* and *b*

    e. *a*, *b*, and *c*

72. Angina pectoris

    a. is a thin, linear muscle in the chest beneath the pectoralis minor

    b. is a tumor in the heart muscle

    c. is always a painless episode of cardiac insufficiency

    d. is chest pain caused by a lack of blood flow to the heart muscle

    e. is another term for a heart attack

73. Which statement is composed of only relative contraindications to exercise testing?

    a. resting DBP > 115 mmHg; ventricular aneurysm; third-degree AV block without pacemaker

    b. fixed-rate pacemaker; mononucleosis; advanced pregnancy

    c. chronic infectious disease; acute infection; moderate valvular heart disease

    d. unstable angina; thrombophlebitis; significant emotional distress

74. To adhere to the principle of specificity, which exercise should be employed by a volleyball player who wants to improve vertical-jump ability?

    a. barbell squats

    b. seated knee extensions

c. seated leg press

d. seated knee flexion

75. Coronary heart disease is a significant cause of death in patients with

a. type 1 diabetes

b. type 2 diabetes

c. syndrome X

d. *a* and *b*

e. *a*, *b*, and *c*

76. What procedure should the fitness professional follow when administering the Cooper 12-minute test of aerobic capacity?

a. Instruct the participant to run, not walk, for the entire test.

b. Instruct the participant to walk, not run, for the entire test.

c. Mark the track by placing marker cones every 40 to 55 yards.

d. Tell the participant that the test is completed when one mile has been covered.

77. To what is the striated appearance of a skeletal muscle fiber due?

a. myofibril arrangements

b. actin and myosin protein filaments

c. overlap of the I band and H zone

d. *a* and *b*

e. *a*, *b*, and *c*

78. When an exercise participant is being positioned on a cycle ergometer, the seat should be adjusted to a height that would allow the knee joint to be in what position when the pedal is at the bottom of the downstroke?

a. straight

b. flexed, approximately 5 degrees

c. flexed, approximately 10 degrees

d. extended, approximately 5 degrees

e. extended, approximately 10 degrees

79. Exercise involving the lactic acid source of energy production generally incorporates what exercise-to-rest ratio?

a. 1:1

b. 1:2

c. 1:3

d. 1:4

e. 1:5

80. Homocysteine levels

a. decrease with age and indicate endothelial dysfunction

b. increase with age and predict mortality in patients with CAD

c. can increase blood viscosity and thrombogenicity

d. *a* and *b*

e. *a*, *b*, and *c*

81. Which of the following statements should you understand before writing a program of exercise at altitude?

a. Endurance performance is severely impaired.

b. Short-term anaerobic performance is not impaired.

c. Sea-level training acclimatizes one for high-altitude training.

d. *a* and *b*

e. *a*, *b*, and *c*

82. The following are events of the excitation-coupling and contraction phases of the sliding filament theory listed randomly. What is the correct order?

a. Muscle fiber is stimulated; action potential travels through the T tubule; Ca^{++} is released from the sarcoplasmic reticulum; Ca^{++} saturates troponin, turning on actin; ATP on the cross-bridge is charged; actomyosin is formed; ATP $\rightarrow$ ADP+ Pi + ENERGY; energy release swivels the cross-bridge; actin slides over myosin.

    b. Muscle fiber is stimulated; Ca^{++} is released from the sarcoplasmic reticulum; action potential travels through the T tubule; Ca^{++} saturates troponin, turning on actin; ATP on the cross-bridge is charged; actomyosin is formed; energy release swivels the cross-bridge; actin slides over myosin; ATP → ADP + Pi + ENERGY.

    c. ATP on the cross-bridge is charged; ATP → ADP + Pi + ENERGY; action potential travels through the T tubule; muscle fiber is stimulated; Ca^{++} is released from the sarcoplasmic reticulum; Ca^{++} saturates troponin, turning on actin; actomyosin is formed; energy release swivels the cross-bridge; actin slides over myosin.

    d. Muscle fiber is stimulated; action potential travels through the T tubule; Ca^{++} saturates troponin, turning on actin; Ca^{++} is released from the sarcoplasmic reticulum; ATP on the cross-bridge is charged; actomyosin is formed; ATP → ADP+ Pi + ENERGY; energy release swivels the cross-bridge; actin slides over myosin.

83. Bone growth during childhood presents a problem(s) because the epiphysis is not united with the bone shaft. Identify the problem(s) from the following list.

    a. Overuse can lead to epiphysitis.

    b. Normal growth may be disrupted.

    c. Calcium content is very low, leading to fractures.

    d. *a* and *b*

    e. *a*, *b*, and *c*

84. What most affects evaporative heat loss during exercise?

    a. ambient temperature

    b. air-current speed

    c. percentage of skin surface exposed to the environment

    d. relative humidity

85. Health counseling skills should include which of the following?

    a. ability to assess readiness for change

    b. ability to assess health-related behaviors

    c. development of a set a values that can be passed on to the patient

d. *a* and *b*

e. *a*, *b*, and *c*

86. How can the strength of contraction in a muscle be graded?

    a. multiple motor unit summation

    b. wave summation

    c. varying the frequency of contraction of individual motor units

    d. *a* and *b*

    e. *a*, *b*, and *c*

87. Which of the following exercises are appropriate for the older adult?

    a. resistance exercises

    b. cardiovascular exercises

    c. balance exercises

    d. *a* and *b*

    e. *a*, *b*, and *c*

88. What is the most important variable in resistance training?

    a. frequency of session per week

    b. amount of resistance

    c. 75 percent from all sources

    d. *a* and *b*

    e. *a*, *b*, and *c*

89. Which of the following abnormal conditions is matched correctly with the appropriate normal symptom?

    a. hypoxia: cessation of breathing

    b. hypoventilation: 12 to 15 breaths per minute

    c. orthostatic hypotension: 120/80 mmHg in a horizontal position

    d. dyspnea: labored breathing

90. A type of training that involves repeated, brief, fast-paced exercise with short rest periods is called

    a. internal training

b. ventilation breakpoint training

c. fartlek training

d. split-sets training

91. Compared to leg work, arm work demonstrates what types of SBP and DBP values?

    a. higher systolic values; lower diastolic values

    b. no differences in systolic values; no differences in diastolic values

    c. high systolic values; higher diastolic values

    d. higher systolic values; no differences in diastolic values

92. You have a client who wishes to exercise aerobically for her health and enjoyment. Which of the following do you prescribe for her?

    a. frequency = 3 times per week

    b. intensity = hard enough to increase breathing, but not hard enough to make you breathless or exhausted

    c. time = 60 minutes

    d. *a* and *b*

    e. *a*, *b*, and *c*

93. The object of most community health and fitness organizations is

    a. to reduce health care costs in the community

    b. to provide a variety of services to the community

    c. to generate a profit

    d. to raise the level of fitness within the community

94. Given the following information, what is the energy cost for a bench-stepping exercise? Step height = 15 centimeters; step rate = 20 steps per minute; weight of subject = 55 kilograms.

    a. 3.91 METs; 3.76 kcal/min

    b. 4.7 METs; 4.6 kcal/min

    c. 4.8 METs; 16.73 ml/kg/min

    d. 5.8 METs; 4.8 kcal/min

95. Given the following information, what is the energy cost for leg cycle ergometry exercise? Work rate = 600 kg/min (100 watts); weight of subject = 50 kilograms.

 a. 7.20 METs; 6.87 kcal/min

 b. 7.61 METs; 7.33 kcal/min

 c. 8.6 METs; 7.5 kcal/min

 d. 8.86 METs; 27.50 ml/kg/min

96. What is the energy cost for a 170-pound, 21-year-old male walking on a treadmill at 90 m/min up a 12 percent grade?

 a. 3.6 METs; 3.1 kcal/min

 b. 3.6 METs; 3.6 kcal/kg/hr

 c. 9.12 METs; 8.0 kcal/kg/hr

 d. 9.13 METs; 12.46 kcal/min

97. What is the energy cost for a 125-pound, 35-year-old female running at 90 m/min up a 10 percent grade on a treadmill?

 a. 8.46 METs; 8.41 kcal/min

 b. 9.1 METs; 7.2 kcal/min

 c. 8.46 METs; 22.03 ml/kg/min

 d. 9.1 METs; 7.4 kcal/kg/hr

98. Given the following information, what is the energy cost of horizontal running? Distance = 10 kilometers; time = 60 minutes; weight of subject = 50 kilograms.

 a. 10.5 METs; 6.1 kcal/min

 b. 10.5 METs; 11.1 kcal/kg/hr

 c. 10.5 METs; 10.7 kcal/kg/hr

 d. 10.5 METs; 9.2 kcal/min

99. Given the following information, what is the energy cost of graded running? Speed = 100 m/min; grade = 10 percent; weight of subject = 50 kilograms.

 a. 9.23 METs; 32.5 ml/kg/min

 b. 9.23 METs; 8.1 kcal/min

 c. 9.2 METs; 10.4 kcal/kg/hr

 d. *a* and *b*

 e. *a*, *b*, and *c*

100. A 45-year-old, 125-pound female exercised on an arm cycle ergometer at 100 watts. What was her energy cost for this activity?

    a. 10.05 METs; 10 kcal/min

    b. 35.17 ml/kg/min

    c. 600 kcal/hr

    d. *a* and *b*

    e. *a*, *b*, and *c*

101. A 200-pound male exercised on a bicycle ergometer for 20 minutes at 60 watts. What was his energy cost?

    a. 25,691 milliliters O_2

    b. 128.5 kcal

    c. 4.2 kcal/kg/hr

    d. *a* and *b*

    e. *a*, *b*, and *c*

102. What is the energy cost for a 23-year-old, 156-pound male running on a level treadmill at 6 mph?

    a. 10.19 METs

    b. 35.66 ml/kg/min

    c. 12.64 kcal/min

    d. *a* and *b*

    e. *a*, *b*, and *c*

103. A 125-pound female pedals a Monark cycle ergometer at 50 rev/min against a resistance of 3.0 kilograms. What is the power output? What is her relative $\dot{V}O_2$?

    a. 900 kgm/m; 35.21 ml/kg/min

    b. 900 kgm/m; 227.5 ml O_2/min

    c. 600 kgm/m; 1998.5 ml/kg/min

    d. 600 kgm/m; 1998.5 milliliters

104. The rating of perceived exertion (RPE) is a reliable indicator of

    a. exercise intensity

    b. exercise tolerance

    c. exercise threshold

d. *a* and *b*

e. *a*, *b*, and *c*

105. The regulatory calcium binding contractile protein of striated muscle is

    a. troponin

    b. tropomyosin

    c. actin

    d. myosin

106. What is the order for muscle fiber recruitment?

    a. SO, FOG, FG

    b. FOG, SO, FG

    c. SO, FG, FOG

    d. FG, SO, FOG

107. Which energy system provides the most rapid source of ATP?

    a. oxidative phosphorylation

    b. anaerobic glycolysis

    c. aerobic glycolysis

    d. ATP-PC

108. Detraining follows which of the following principles?

    a. overtraining

    b. overload

    c. reversibility

    d. specificity

109. Which of the following should be considered when selecting an appropriate exercise intensity for a client?

    a. level of fitness

    b. medications

    c. individual program objectives

    d. *a* and *b*

    e. *a*, *b*, and *c*

110. Which of the following statements accurately define *progressive resistance?*

    a. a gradual cycling of specificity, intensity, and volume of training

    b. Motor units are generally activated on the basis of a fixed order during training.

    c. Training stimulus must be progressively increased during training.

    d. training for more than one sport at the same time

111. Using and adjusting RPE during exercise are easy and effective. Which of the following are true about RPE?

    a. RPE coincides with objectives of physiologic and metabolic strain.

    b. An RPE of 13 or 14 (exercise that feels "somewhat" hard) coincides with about 7 percent HR max during treadmill exercise.

    c. An RPE of 11 to 12 corresponds to the lactate threshold in trained and untrained individuals.

    d. *a* and *b*

    e. *a*, *b*, and *c*

CASE STUDY

Lynn is a 52-year-old vice president of a large company. She is 66 inches tall, weighs 140 pounds, and smokes one pack of cigarettes a day. She has a resting HR of 80 bpm and 35 percent body fat. Her blood chemistry values are TC = 280 mg/dl; HDL-C = 30 mg/dl, and LDL-C = 146 mg/dl. Lynn's mother died of a heart attack at the age of 63 and her father died of a heart attack at the age of 67. You perform a submaximal bicycle ergometer test and obtain the following data:

Stage	Work rate (kgm · min⁻¹)	HR (min 2)	HR (min 3)
1	150	118	120
2	300	134	136

Pedal rate = 50 rpm; predicted HR max = 182 bpm; HR max = 155 bpm.
Reprinted from Howley and Franks, 1997.

112. What does Lynn's blood profile indicate?
    a. TC is high.
    b. LDL-C is a positive risk factor for CAD.
    c. TC : HDL-C ratio is approximately 3.9.
    d. *a* and *b*
    e. *a*, *b*, and *c*

113. What is Lynn's $\dot{V}O_2$ at the end of stage 2?
    a. 14. 9 ml/kg/min: 4.26 METs
    b. 15.5 ml/kg/min: 4.43 METs
    c. 16.0 ml/kg/min: 4.57 METs
    d. 16.5 ml/kg/min: 4.71 METs

114. Lynn wishes to reduce her body fat to 23 percent. What would be her corresponding target body weight?
    a. 137.1 lb
    b. 124.7 lb
    c. 61.2 kg
    d. 62.3 kg

115. Overall, what is revealed by Lynn's medical history?
    a. a need to participate in a smoking cessation program
    b. a positive health history for CAD
    c. a need to raise HDL-C and lower LDL-C
    d. *a* and *b*
    e. *a*, *b*, and *c*

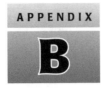

Practice Examination Blank Score Sheet

Appendix B contains a blank score sheet for the practice examination. For each question, there is a blank space where you can write the answer and another blank space where you can write the correct answer to questions you have missed. This will make it much easier for you to review those questions you answered incorrectly. Also included is a column in which to enter the KSA with which each answer corresponds. Note that this blank score sheet does not mirror the score sheet used during the actual exam. For the actual exam you will be asked to use a scan sheet.

Your question #	Correct answer	KSA # answer	Category
1			
2			
3			
4			
5			
6			
7			
8			
9			

Your question #	Correct answer	KSA # answer	Category
10			
11			
12			
13			
14			
15			
16			
17			
18			
19			
20			
21			
22			
23			
24			
25			
26			
27			
28			
29			
30			
31			
32			
33			

Your question #	Correct answer	KSA # answer	Category
34			
35			
36			
37			
38			
39			
40			
41			
42			
43			
44			
45			
46			
47			
48			
49			
50			
51			
52			
53			
54			
55			
56			
57			

Your question #	Correct answer	KSA # answer	Category
58			
59			
60			
61			
62			
63			
64			
65			
66			
67			
68			
69			
70			
71			
72			
73			
74			
75			
76			
77			
78			
79			
80			
81			

Your question #	Correct answer	KSA # answer	Category
82			
83			
84			
85			
86			
87			
88			
89			
90			
91			
92			
93			
94			
95			
96			
97			
98			
99			
100			
101			
102			
103			
104			
105			

Your question #	Correct answer	KSA # answer	Category
106			
107			
108			
109			
110			
111			
112			
113			
114			
115			

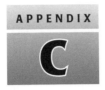

Answers to the Practice Examination

Sequential list of answers

1. b	2. a	3. b	4. b	5. b
6. c	7. c	8. b	9. c	10. e
11. a	12. c	13. c	14. b	15. b
16. a	17. b	18. a	19. a	20. a
21. d	22. a	23. d	24. b	25. d
26. d	27. e	28. b	29. e	30. b
31. d	32. b	33. d	34. d	35. d
36. a	37. d	38. e	39. b	40. d
41. e	42. b	43. e	44. b	45. e
46. d	47. b	48. d	49. a	50. a
51. c	52. d	53. d	54. c	55. e
56. e	57. b	58. c	59. e	60. e
61. d	62. d	63. e	64. d	65. a
66. d	67. e	68. d	69. b	70. b
71. d	72. d	73. b	74. a	75. e
76. c	77. d	78. b	79. b	80. b

81. d	82. d	83. b	84. d	85. d
86. e	87. e	88. b	89. b	90. a
91. c	92. d	93. b	94. a	95. b
96. d	97. a	98. d	99. e	100. e
101. e	102. e	103. a	104. d	105. a
106. a	107. d	108. c	109. e	110. c
111. e	112. d	113. b	114. c	115. e

ANSWERS TO THE PRACTICE EXAMINATION BY KSA CATEGORY

In this section, we have listed the answers to the practice questions according to KSA category. After taking and grading your practice examination, you can mark the questions that you did not answer correctly and write in the corresponding KSA. This will help give you an accurate picture of your strengths and weaknesses.

Anatomy and Biomechanics—8				
11. a	21. d	31. d	40. d	49. a
57. b	64. d	71.d		
Exercise Physiology—21				
1. b	2. a	12. c	22. a	32. b
41. e	42. b	50. a	58. c	65. a
72. d	77. d	82. d	86. e	89. b
91. c	104. d	105. a	106. a	107. d
108. c				

Human Development and Aging—8

3. b	13. c	23. d	53. d	60. e
67. e	83. e	87. e		

Pathophysiology and Risk Factors—10

6. c	16. a	26. d	35. d	44. b
52. d	62. d	69. b	75. e	80. b

Human Behavior and Psychology—5

4. b	14. b	24. b	33. d	85. d

Health Appraisal and Fitness Testing—10

5. b	15. b	25. d	34. d	43. e
51. c	59. e	66. d	73. b	78. b

Safety, Injury Prevention, and Emergency Care—5

7. c	17. b	27. e	36. a	45. e

Exercise Programming—22

8. b	18. a	28. b	37. d	46. d
54. c	61. d	63. e	68. d	70. b
74. a	76. c	79. b	81. d	84. d
88. b	90. a	92. d	93. b	109. e
110. c	111. e			

Nutrition and Weight Management—6

9. c	19. a	29. e	38. e	47. b
55. e				

Program Administration and Management—6

10. e	20. a	30. b	39. b	48. d
56. e				

Metabolic Equations—10				
94. a	95. b	96. d	97. a	98. d
99. e	100. e	101. e	102. e	103. a
Case Study—4				
112. d	113. b	114. c	115. e	

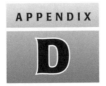

APPENDIX

D

Practice Examination Profile Sheet

Use this profile sheet to determine the percentage of questions you answered correctly for each KSA category and for the entire practice exam. Use the following steps to determine your score.

Step One: After finishing the practice exam, use appendix C to score your exam. Mark all incorrect responses by placing the correct answer in the space provided.

Step Two: For each incorrect response, note its corresponding KSA category by placing a tally mark in the appropriate KSA category tally column on the profile sheet. Subtract your tally from the maximum score for the KSA to derive your score. Divide your score by the maximum score to derive the percentage of correct responses for each KSA category. We suggest marking any KSA category below 75% as an area needing further study.

Step Three: To calculate your overall test score, simply total the column labeled "Your Score" and divide this sum by the total number of test questions—115. Remember, in order to receive certification, you will need to score about 70% (according to current standards). Please note, while you will receive 115 questions on the actual exam, fifteen questions are not counted and are designed for statistical sampling only.

KSA category	Tally	Maximum score	Your score	Percent correct	Check categories in need of improvement
Anatomy and Biomechanics		8			
Exercise Physiology		21			
Human Development and Aging		8			
Pathophysiology and Risk Factors		10			
Human Behavior and Psychology		5			
Health Appraisal and Fitness Testing		10			
Safety, Injury Prevention, and Emergency Care		5			
Exercise Programming		22			
Nutrition and Weight Management		6			
Program Administration and Management		6			
Metabolic Equations		10			
Case Studies		4			
Totals		**115**			

About the Authors

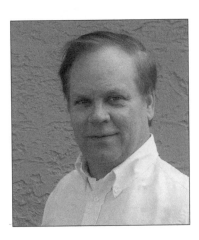

Larry D. Isaacs is a professor and directs the activities of the exercise biology program at Wright State University in Dayton, Ohio. He has worked at the university since 1979, teaching both undergraduate and graduate students in courses covering clinical exercise physiology, exercise prescription, motor development, motor learning, and research methods. He is responsible for developing the school's exercise biology/pre-physical therapy/pre-medical program within the department of biological sciences.

Isaacs received his PhD from the University of Maryland in 1979. His areas of concentration included clinical exercise physiology, motor development, physiological growth and development, research and statistics, and administration. A prolific writer, Isaacs is the author or coauthor of 15 other books and numerous scholarly articles. He is a research fellow of the American Alliance for Health, Physical Education, Recreation and Dance, and he is a member of the American College of Sports Medicine, with whom he is certified as a Health/Fitness Instructor.

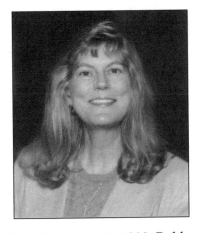

Roberta L. Pohlman is an associate professor of biological sciences at Wright State University. She has been at the university since 1984 and has done research and taught undergraduate and graduate classes in all areas of exercise science. With Isaacs, she helped in the development of the exercise biology program. Pohlman is certified as an exercise test technologist by the American College of Sports Medicine (ACSM). After receiving her PhD in exercise physiology from Ohio State University in 1982, Pohlman went on to complete a two-year postdoctoral fellowship in research at St. Louis University Medical School. She is a coauthor of one other book. She has also served on the editorial advisory committee for *Future Focus*, a journal of the Ohio Association for Health, Physical Education and Recreation, and on the editorial review boards for *Strategies* and *JOHPERD*, which are both journals of the American Alliance for Health, Physical Education, Recreation and Dance. Pohlman is a member of both ACSM and the American Physiological Society.

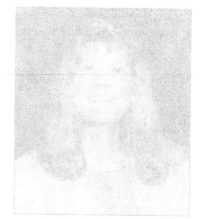